OKANAGAN UNIV/COLLEGE LIBRARY

S0-AUL-206

WITHDRAWN

Ethical Dilemmas in Assisted Reproduction

COLLEGE
LIBRARY
BRITISH COLUMBIA

STUDIES IN PROFERTILITY SERIES

VOLUME 7

Ethical Dilemmas in Assisted Reproduction

EDITED BY F. SHENFIELD AND C. SUREAU

*The publication of this book has been made possible
by an educational grant from NV Organon*

The Parthenon Publishing Group
International Publishers in Medicine, Science & Technology

NEW YORK   LONDON

Published in the USA by
The Parthenon Publishing Group Inc.
One Blue Hill Plaza
PO Box 1564, Pearl River,
New York 10965, USA

Published in the UK by
The Parthenon Publishing Group Limited
Casterton Hall, Carnforth,
Lancs LA6 2LA, UK

Copyright © 1997 Parthenon Publishing Group

Library of Congress Cataloging-in-Publication Data
Ethical dilemmas in assisted reproduction/edited by F. Shenfield and C. Sureau.
    p.   cm. — (Studies in profertility series; v. 7)
    Includes bibliographical references and index.
    ISBN 1-85070-916-5
    1. Human reproductive technology—Moral and ethical aspects.
I. Shenfield, F.   II. Sureau, Claude.   III. Series.
RG133.5.E838   1997
176—dc21   97-19650
                                                                                  CIP

British Library Cataloguing in Publication Data
Ethical dilemmas in assisted reproduction. – (Studies in profertility series; v. 7)
    1. Human reproductive technology – Moral and ethical aspects
    I. Shenfield, F.   II. Sureau, Claude
    176

    ISBN 1-85070-916-5

First published 1997

*No part of this book may be reproduced
in any form without permission from the publishers except for the
quotation of brief passages for the purposes of review.*

Composition by AMA Graphics Ltd., Preston, UK
Printed and bound by Butler & Tanner Ltd., London and Frome, UK

Contents

List of contributors

P. R. Brinsden
Bourn Hall Clinic
Bourn
Cambridge CB3 7TR
UK

B. M. Dickens
Faculty of Law
University of Toronto
84 Queen's Park Crescent
Toronto
Ontario
Canada M5S 2C5

R. G. Edwards
Churchill College
Cambridge
UK

V. English
Medical Ethics
British Medical Association
BMA House
Tavistock Square
London WC1H 9PJ
UK

M. Jones
Department of Obstetrics and
  Gynaecology
University of Western Ontario
London, Ontario
Canada

G. M. Lockwood
Green College
University of Oxford
Woodstock Road
Oxford
UK

J. Milliez
Clinical Obstetrics and Gynecology
Hopital St. Antoine
184 rue du Faubourg St. Antoine
75012 Paris Cedex 12
France

I. Nisand
Gynécologie Obstétrique et
  Biologie de la Reproduction
Université Paris V–Rene Descartes
  CHU Ouest
78 303 Poissy-Cedex
France

J. A. Nisker
Department of Obstetrics and
  Gynaecology
University Hospital
339 Windermere Road
London, Ontario N6A 5A5
Canada

C. Ramogida
Association Pauline et Adrien
920 Chemin du Pre Seigneur
Villennes s/Seine 78250
France

F. Shenfield
Reproductive Medicine Unit
University College London Medical
  School
Obstetrics Hospital
Huntley Street
London WC1 6AE
UK

A. Sommerville
40 Egremont Road
London SE27 08H
UK

C. Sureau
Institut Théramex
Bioéthique
Santé de la Femme et Société
38–40 av de New York
75768 Paris Cedex 16
France

H. Tournaye
Center for Reproductive Medicine
University Hospital
Brussels Free University
101 Laarbeeklaan
B-1090 Brussels
Belgium

A. Van Steirteghem
Center for Reproductive Medicine
University Hospital
Brussels Free University
101 Laarbeeklaan
B-1090 Brussels
Belgium

Introduction: The modern ethical practice of assisted human conception

R. G. Edwards

It is a privilege to read the various contributions to this small book. Its contents show that it could well prove to have an importance far greater than its comparative size. It deals with the ethics of assisted human reproduction, as it delves deeply into traditions of ethics and law in modern societies. *In vitro* fertilization (IVF) and other recent advances have enlarged the immense number of social, ethical and legal issues associated with human conception, widening the age-old arguments on contraception and abortion to new and more complex fields. Straightforward IVF was enough to set up an immense hullaballoo about morals and science in the 1970s and 1980s, and the ethical complexities of many issues raised by this procedure, such as gamete donation or surrogacy, remain with us today. As we now approach the millennium, its new developments raise ever-more social problems as possibilities of interference with genetic systems or new embryological methods enter the arena.

The scale and width of these issues must be apparent to anyone who scans the daily newspapers or glances at television news: a near-daily fare of fresh reproductive items usually listed as pioneering advances. To be true, most of the underlying opportunities for novel forms of conception have been with us for 10 or more years by now. But the ethics have hardly kept in touch, and, for some reason or other, the role of voluntary or professional bodies has been down-graded in favor of legislation as country after country introduces or proposes restrictive law to cover one item after another. And, of course, legislation once passed is a lethargic animal, unwilling to change, dominated by the wording of individual clauses in Acts of Parliament or long-accepted, outdated principles. Law, lawyers and sociologists replace doctors, scientists and counsellors in determining acceptable clinical practice, and decide what can or cannot be done without ever sitting in front of a single patient whose life and hopes they govern.

There are compensations for we professionals working in this field of medicine. The sheer insistence and unexpected reactions of patients facing their own particular problems are a source of constant inspiration to investigators trying to find delicate and acceptable solutions to complex issues. We have witnessed in the past week a Philippino woman of 63 insisting to her IVF doctor that she was only 50, and so being helped to produce a newborn baby at this fine age. We must not condone untruths, but she has helped to make medical history, and her own mother was overjoyed when told about her unexpected new grandchild! There are other such examples, of an XO patient who became the first woman with secondary amenorrhea to deliver a child via oocyte donation, IVF and hormone replacement therapy. There was the South African mother who was the first to enable her daughter to have children by carrying them to full term in her own uterus. What sort of terms can be applied to situations such as this, which would never have been permitted to go ahead under the repressive legislation passed in many countries? Perhaps we should learn to use terms such as 'love' to describe such outstanding altruism, a word seldom read in ethical or legal tracts.

Many of the newer issues, and some of those which have been with us for a decade or more, are covered in this book. A constant background issue since IVF, and perhaps ovulation induction began, has concerned the rights or privileges of infertile patients to receive State support for their treatment. There are dangers of an economic selection of patients for fertility treatments when national funds allotted for this purpose are very limited, as in the UK. In this book, Dr Shenfield addresses the provision of State funding to characteristics in the patient, such as marital status, age, and the number of children the patient already has. Those who are unmarried, old, and already have four children shall not receive State and other benefits. This is an argument about resources rather than IVF, and it shows once again how the rich reap the benefits from most new forms of novel clinical treatments.

The ethics of gamete donation inspires the authors of two chapters, with further comments in the Conclusion. Dr Shenfield and Professor Sureau write about counselling sperm donors, and comment that the word 'donor' implies gift with no payment. The relation between donor, recipients and child is exceedingly complex. Many donors do not object to providing identifying information and expect no financial reward. They are owed duties by the provider and the recipient, and are sometimes very hard to find. Advertisements and payments are considered bad form. The motivation of donors can sometimes be complex, and may include psychological attitudes stemming from the termination of their own partnership, an impression of being unwanted as a child or even a feeling of a debt to life. Dr Lockwood discusses oocyte donation, and how the birth mother is the legal mother under English law. A wide range of women could benefit from this procedure, and numbers who could be helped become even larger as new technologies are introduced. Donation must be altruistic according to the Human Fertilisation and Embryology Authority (HFEA). Yet various classes of donors exist, from unpaid unrelated altruistic donors to those who share their oocytes as they undergo their own gamete intra-fallopian transfer (GIFT) or IVF. The gold standard of altruism fails to provide enough donors in most societies, especially since some of them stipulate who shall receive their oocytes. Commercial donation is the least regarded, yet these donors often have various advantages in relation to oocyte donation. They have no interest or desire to keep the child, hand it over without hesitation, do not question who should receive their oocytes, and do not have a partner who himself needs counselling. Indeed, we are currently witnessing strong debates within our profession about differing attitudes to commerce and altruism, and even strong self-doubts in some doctors about a rampant commercialism in gamete donation and surrogate parenting.

Surrogate parenting has indeed raised more than its equal share of ethical arguments – sometimes in almost angry debates in Parliament or during protracted legal cases. Ms English and her colleagues show how parliamentary attitudes to the procedure have changed from near horror as the first case emerged, to the present practice of Parliamentary provisions of parental orders for transferring parentage from surrogate to intended parents, an increased medical involvement and even notions of public funding. Many aspects of the treatment are regulated by the UK Human Fertilisation and Embryology Authority. The frequency and complexity of some consequences of surrogacy, such as the surrogate keeping the baby, are being defined more clearly as practice steadily expands. This particular problem is relatively small in numbers but a major headache in law. Perhaps an increased openness about the procedure and its benefits has reduced the risks of misuse.

Embryo reduction, with its consequentialist background of balancing benefits and risks, has become widely practised. Sometimes it is impossible to avoid highly multiple pregnancies, such as when some small follicles do not show up on ultrasound during ovarian stimulation. On other occasions, the careless use of intercourse or insemination when too many follicles are identified, or the replacement of a large number of embryos, inevitably lead to multiple pregnancies. The subsequent need for embryo reduction with triplets or higher multiple pregnancies is discussed by Professor Nisand and Dr Shenfield, who examine the treatment in the context of a conflict between the interests of the mothers and of the 'fetal siblings'. The obstetric advantages of reduction are overwhelming, but so are the risks and ethical difficulties, such as accidental abortion, the ethical difficulties in selecting which fetuses to abort and controversy about reducing multiple pregnancies to twins or singletons. There is also a wide clinical disagreement about reducing twins to singletons.

Sex selection is a matter related to fetal reduction. It raises an especially poignant form of the balance between a mother's rights and the value of human fetal life throughout pregnancy. Professor Nisker discusses sex selection as practised in a clinic on the US/Canadian border, in a somewhat droll but telling manner. Many Canadian women migrate to this clinic in a small town south of the US border in the hope of having a selective termination of their female fetuses. The need for Canadian couples to go to the USA for this treatment is revealing in itself, and emphasizes the problems existing in Canada for those who wish to use this method for sex control. In this example, three distinct sets of values converge, Canadian, USA and South Asian. The South Asian problem originates with immigrants from India, where the social problems associated with girls are well known. Professor Nisker covers all these complexities of the situation, comparing differing social values, and legal and professional standards in dealing with this intractable aspect of human conception.

Research on embryos has always attracted considerable ethical attention in the past, and will continue to do so in the future. It poses a literally insolvable difference in attitudes between those who believe that life and the soul begin at fertilization and those who totally reject these beliefs. Whether research should be done at all is therefore the first question to be answered, since many moral theologians consider that human life begins at fertilization and must be protected. Some countries have expressed no doubts that such research must be done, to improve the health of their citizens. In these countries, the first cleavage division, the onset of embryonic transcription, implantation or day 14 have all been considered as establishing a good balance between the need for research and the protection of meaningful human life. UK law permits the establishment of embryos for research, to a limit of day 14, while German law seems to be based on totipotency of blastomeres. Dr Shenfield and Professor Sureau describe these complex aspects, describing the necessity for embryo research in relation and according to legislation in various countries. They point out the benefits to be gained for many patients, the inconsistencies in some parliamentary decisions, and the consequences of various lines of action; they have cogently summarized the complex arguments of the past and some of the future. Perhaps it should be stressed that the huge loss of human embryos before implantation negates any concept of the soul entering the egg at fertilization, and that research could well lessen this enormous rate of loss.

New developments coming on-stream in IVF clinics include the avoidance of inherited disease by diagnosing it in preimplantation embryos, and the alleviation of male infertility by the use of the intracytoplasmic injection of a single spermatozoon. Professor Milliez and Dr Sureau discuss preimplantation diagnosis including the analysis of aneuploidy in embryos of older women, germline therapy and other forms of interference into the genetic constitution of gametes and embryos. This area of investigation is regarded by some people as an agenda for eugenics rather than a vehicle for family planning, but the authors have a wider and more liberal approach to the treatments as being part of preventive medicine. The problems of follow-up of children conceived by these means are discussed in relation to the intrusion in to the privacy of the family.

Ethical aspects of intracytoplasmic sperm injection are dealt with by Professor Van Steirteghem and his colleagues. The ethical issues here concern professional standards as much as the correct treatment of patients. Treating men with literally 100 or fewer spermatozoa inevitably involves questions about the genetic nature of the disease, its side-effects and the risks to the child. One fascinating genetic situation, recently identified, is the presence of many chromosomal microdeletions which prevent the normal formation of the testis, and are now known to be increasingly involved in other forms of clinical illnesses. This knowledge has opened ethical aspects of a possibly increased level of genetic defects in spermatozoa of men with extreme oligozoospermia, so that potential risks to the child must be balanced with the advantages to the future parents. Fortunately, well-rehearsed screening and counselling protocols have been available to patients, arising from previous work on amnio-centesis and chorionic villus sampling.

The interfaces between assisted reproduction, ethics and law are discussed by Professor Dickens. He stresses that law lacks an ethical dimension, and points out how morally flawed conduct may be acceptable provided the conduct of the investigators and its consequences do not exceed the limits of popular tolerance. Different legal systems interact in various ways with ethics, so that Anglo-Saxon law is based on customary practices within the community, the Napoleonic Code defines rights, and religious law is based on spiritual values. Professional and specialist agencies also set standards in some societies and their decisions may be ratified in law. In general, law may prevail at the cost of ethics, as we have seen in UK this year, e.g. the insistence of the HFEA to destroy 3000 cryopreserved embryos.

Finally, Mme Ramogida provides the patient's point-of-view. This has long been needed, as it describes how countless numbers of men and women trek to IVF and other clinics, searching for the conception they so desperately desire. The chapter is brief but good reading for all that. She challenges the principle of unpaid oocyte donation, comments on the many women travelling abroad for oocyte donation, just as they used to do for abortion, and is certain that no legislation in the world will be able to dictate to parents how to behave to their child conceived by gamete donation. She sums up in a few words what so many patients passionately believe. Her demand that patients' associations claim their rights to partake in decision-making is very long overdue. Let us hope that they are successful.

1

Justice and access to fertility treatments

F. Shenfield

INTRODUCTION

There is a very specific UK dimension concerning the economic picture of fertility treatments: that of a dearth of state-subsidized resources in the face of the demand and need. Not only does it result in economic selection, as some treatments will be restricted to the wealthier sections of the population, but also inherently in a double-pronged iniquity. This stems from the lack of central government policy on infertility treatment, which fails to state a minimum level to be purchased, and the variable access to therapy from region to region.

There are several implications at society level. In particular, it affects the primary social unit encompassing the couple wishing to enlarge their family when, for instance, their age and status are taken into consideration. The secondary effect, on society at large, is in the realm of economics. One may wish, as a deontologist, to treat every patient with the best possible appropriate treatment, regardless of cost. As doctors, we are not trained to be economists, nor is it our vocational call, otherwise indeed we would not be practising in our chosen field. But we are part of society as well, with its watchdogs telling us about scarce resources, cost effectiveness, demand and supply.

From the ethical point of view, the imbalance between supply and demand, and funding to care for the demand (or clinical need if we replace economic jargon by terms that we medical practitioners are more used to handling), we face a problem of justice, as to whom is selected as deserving of subsidized treatment, and a problem of policy, as to who may decide on this access to treatment. There is, of course, very little distance between policy and politics, and indeed it was a political post-war decision to create the National Health Service (NHS) in the UK, based on the ideal of equal access to treatment for all citizens in need. In order to understand the basis of the present unequal access of British infertile couples to subsidized State treatment, it is essential initially to address the mechanics of NHS provisions.

PROVISION AND ECONOMICS

Since the recent reforms of the NHS Act[2] applied in the General Medical Services Regulations 1992[3], which have modified the 1977 Act[4], the disparity of provision in the UK has been extensively discussed[5]. This affects particularly 'assisted' techniques in fertility treatment, the cost of which private insurance companies do not cover in the UK. The reforms have introduced an 'internal market' with acquirers (or purchasers) and providers. This applies to specialist services, of which fertility treatment is one.

A District Health Authority (DHA) enters into contracts with DHA managed units, called 'trusts', but, according to legislation (S4 (3)), these are not to give rise to contractual rights and liabilities. There are special conciliation mechanisms, and arbitration is possible by the Secretary of State, who delegates powers first to Area Health Authorities (AHAs), then Regional and then District Health Authorities. The lack of central policy on provision of fertility services from the Department of Health level places immediate obstacles in the path of infertile couples.

The need for specialist fertility treatments is undeniable and quantifiable: estimation of necessary resources[6,7] is based on the incidence of infertility in the population, with a prevalence (or proportion of women at any point in time experiencing subfertility) of 9–14%. The need and provision for *in vitro* fertilization (IVF), a complex form of infertility treatment, now almost 20 years old and most often purchased through a specific contract, may be used as an example of the hiatus between need and provision which exists in the NHS. It is seen by purchasers as a 'costly' treatment per unit provided, although several papers have demonstrated its 'cost effectiveness' per cycle when clinically indicated, as indeed, if compared for instance with difficult tubal surgery which is unlikely to succeed. The need for IVF is estimated as being 100 IVF cycles per year for each 250 000 population (or 40 cycles per 100 000). Recent reports published over the last 2 years and commissioned by the patients' support group, the National Infertility Awareness Campaign, into the state of provision of fertility services in the country, show that 8.1 cycles per 100 000 were funded in 1994/1995[8]. This compares with the estimated need of 40, resulting in a comparative lack of 32.9 cycles per 100 000 population. This figure was calculated in response to a questionnaire, with a 74% rate of return.

In contrast, there is relatively less shortfall in the total number of cycles performed in the UK, as compared to the need: 20 213 cycles were performed in the year 1994[9], in the face of an estimated need for 22 000 cycles (estimation based on a UK population of 55 million). The salient feature, however, is the fact that the proportion of private/NHS provision in IVF is still of the order of 80% private to 20% NHS. The same National Survey found that, by 1995, 35% of health authorities funded no treatments, 11% funded 15–30 cycles and only 4% funded 30 or more. Scotland came nearest to providing for the estimated needs of the local population. Some areas (51%) have been coping with restrictions in budget allocations to fertility treatments by introducing 'eligibility criteria' for couples to access their provision in infertility treatment; 91% of those related to an upper limit for the woman's age; 89% to the number of previous children and 71% to previous cycles already undertaken. This unfair selection is also sexist, as the male partner's age is hardly ever taken into consideration. But, of course, the main problem is that the treatment of an older female is less likely to succeed, whilst the age of the male partner has very little bearing on success rates (a cost–benefit analysis of a financial kind).

Thus, in the UK, the economic position of a couple intrinsically influences access to fertility treatment. This is to be contrasted with the positions in France and Germany where four cycles of IVF may be subsidized by the health system. Other relatively expensive treatments like ovulation induction with gonadotropins, for instance, are also affected. Another salient example is the relative unavailability of intracytoplasmic sperm injection on the NHS. Finally, an important detail is that a majority of health authorities said they would welcome national guidelines for provision of treatments, as some decisions are sometimes made purely on the grounds of local availability. This is another (psychologically) onerous demand on a manager, and yet it should be a clinical decision to treat or not for any disease, including infertility.

OTHER SOCIOECONOMIC FACTORS OF RESTRICTION

Let us analyze further the means of selection for treatment used by several Health Authorities. They are the above-mentioned 'eligibility criteria' or arbitrary limits imposed on patients who need 'assisted' fertility treatments. The marital status of the couple, or the number of children already under their care may be factors considered. In France, the legislation on assisted reproduction[10] states that available treatment is restricted to couples 'married or living together for 2 years', whilst there is no such provision in the UK Act.

Age is another factor used as a limit to access, usually that of the female half of the couple. The French legislation also makes clear that a limit is expected (un couple 'en age de se reproduire'), but talks about the couple's age being 'reproductive age'; implying rather than specifying the physiological inequality which nature imposes on the male and female in terms of aging gametes. Taking account of the 'welfare of the child', which is a statutory requirement in the UK, is a factor often invoked in this argument. It is stated that a relevant factor is the amount of time parents would be alive to look after the resulting child. It would, however, be fairer to use a joint upper limit for the added ages of both prospective parents rather than to concentrate on the age of the female only. This particular criterion is sometimes used ruthlessly. In October 1994, the High Court upheld the decision of a District Health Authority not to provide publicly funded treatment for a woman of 36, who had been several years on a NHS waiting list for IVF and who was removed from the list when she had reached the age of 35 years.

The discussion in Court revolved primarily on what constitutes a 'reasonable use of public resources'. The patient concerned has now been delivered of a healthy child, thanks to the generosity of an anonymous benefactor who paid for private IVF treatment after reading of her plight in the lay press. This particular selection, however, is rationalized on the grounds of cost effectiveness, as success decreases with female age. A final comment on how effectiveness is measured will bring me to my concluding remarks in the realm of ethics, and a brief discussion on justice in a state-provided health-care system where there is a finite amount of resources.

CONCLUSION

The problem of access to and selection for fertility treatments in the UK is particularly relevant to several current issues which have led to debates about the funding of health systems in general. The provocative title of 'Rationing is now accepted as inevitable by all sides' was only one of many in the recent medical press[11]. It has been argued that it is a debate which should not be confused with this 'over-effectiveness and funding of the NHS', and, as much as the first part of the statement seems obvious, the second is arguably less so. Funding of the NHS is a political decision, one which should be exercising public debate when submitted to guidance from the Treasury. The facts that a rationing agenda group has been formed, and that 'Being creative about rationing' makes the title of yet another *British Medical Journal* leader[12], are a symptom either of acceptance of the process, or an attempt to waken those who have not realized the pervasiveness of the problems in all fields of health supply.

We will nevertheless confine our remarks to the field of fertility, although, of all the chapters, this is the least specific to our specialized field.

The allocation of resources 'on the basis of needs with an eye to cost-effectiveness' has been branded as benign but unhelpful by one of the most considerate and leading thinkers in medical ethics. He applies the 'veil of ignorance' theory of Rawls[13] to people's predispositions, and endows them with information and the ability to make rational decisions in a world where wealth is justly distributed (in an egalitarian manner). This proposed model takes age into account with a bias against the elderly, who have already 'had their innings'. We observe that, in our field, patients are relatively young; furthermore, no one has ever quantified the 'value' of youth to society, even in simple economic terms, as the future providers for their elders' pensions. Thus, does this proposed model stand better for our fertility patients than the classical models which are so prone to frailty?

Let us examine in turn some of the classical ethical theories as applied to infertility.

The utilitarian view

If one assumes that available resources are organized in such a way that, when available, the treatment is at least used effectively[14], let us pretend that it is morally right to define cost-effectiveness only in market economy terms, using a successful pregnancy as a marker. It may then be logical to reserve costly treatments like IVF to those who have a higher chance of success in terms of 'take home baby rate', i.e. the younger age group.

In a utilitarian manner, the happiness of more people can be added up, enhancing total happiness in society, and at least all people of a certain age (i.e. women under the age of 35, for instance) are counted as equal, another tenet of the utilitarian theory[15]. The main objection to this is that it condones in practice the inequality of success opportunity, especially for women over the age of 35–37 (the limit often used), rendering all older couples very much unequal in the face of their fertility problem. Furthermore, another dimension is totally ignored, that of the therapeutic role of trying to help a couple who might have a realistically poor chance of a 'take home baby'. In other words, success of fertility treatment may not only be considered in terms of live birth rate. There is another benefit, that of coming to terms with infertility, which pertains to 'failed' treatment, along with the concomitant counselling, the importance of which the UK legislation rightly stresses[16].

The utilitarian argument thus fails to give a satisfactory reason for limiting access to IVF in view of age, or rather utilitarian theory is distorted in order to condone mercantile selection on a financially biased short-term criterion – the live-baby-rate per treatment. Consequentialist theory, often used in the debate about the distribution of scarce resources in order to maximize the beneficial outcome for society, may be flawed if the objective is distorted. The alternative view is that consequentialist theories are not wholly suited to the art of medicine, as the objective end-point of benefiting the patient may be measured, thanks to 'evidence-based medicine', but may also be quantified in terms less easily measured than molecules, like relief of distress, well-being and coming to terms with a life crisis.

What about rights?

The place of rights theories in an ethical debate is controversial. According to Ronald Dworkin, 'In most cases when we say that someone has a "right" to do something, we imply that it would be wrong to interfere with his doing it, or at least that some special grounds are needed for justifying any interference'[17]. In other words, rights theories can best be fitted to the politico-legal scene, as rights enable 'agents' to obtain in society what may be morally their due, but has historically escaped them. Rights can also be described as claim rights (or positive) and liberty rights (or negative). Many international conventions and charters, including the European Convention on Human Rights, with the well-known article 12, 'to found a family', 'acknowledge the unacceptability of obstructing someone in the exercise of that right'[18] rather than demanding positive action, like allocation of resources to this particular matter. The need for justice is thus a more powerful argument in this case than the language of rights, but does the duty of care of practitioners include political action on their behalf?

The deontological point of view

This view concerns carers and their duty to patients (of beneficience, non-malevolence and respect of their autonomy, to use three of the four famous principles which, with justice itself, have been found to be wanting even by a well-known proponent[19] because of their propensity to clash). The lack of a tradition of natalist policy may explain the differences between the French and British approaches in terms of provisions for IVF, but the double iniquity represented by the variability between areas compounds the injustice of restricted State funding for adequate provisions.

It may become inevitable that even carers, accustomed as they are to a one-to-one relationship of duty of care, play a larger role in the society in which they practice and become involved in the essence of the *res politica*. This would be most affectively achieved by carers acting in unison, as a profession, and is indeed one of the roles, which includes education both of other practitioners, purchasing agents and the public which professional societies and the patients' self-help groups try to achieve in the face of political obstacles.

FINALLY, WHAT ABOUT JUSTICE?

Whether we consider analysis of justice in terms of needs or deserts is a classical ethical question. That the needs of the UK population in the realm of assisted reproduction treatment in the NHS are not met is obvious from the figures quoted above. The prioritization effected by Area Health Authorities is performed in a haphazard way with wide regional variations. The national survey found that 'Most Area Health Authorities would favor national guidelines on eligibility criteria and the level of IVF to be purchased', indicating their unease at being placed in this judgmental position of selection to access. It also found a gap between authorities which fund to a significant level and the poor providers, without any middle ground. Who can redress this injustice? Is it right that vulnerable patients should have to conduct a political fight, or indeed that their carers should have to do so? Does duty of care encompass political action, rather than treating patients or doing research? In 'What makes a just healthcare system?', Benatar describes some of the features as necessary to this qualification: universal access, access to an 'adequate level of care' and fair distribution of the burdens of rationing care to name those which certainly do not apply to our fertility patients in the UK[20].

To start by implementing those may allow all of our patients to climb 'Rachel's ladder'[21] in a fair and just manner. Even if it cannot be guaranteed to lead to the long awaited pregnancy, it will at least allow a fair trial.

REFERENCES

1. Bull, A. and Lyons, C. (1994). Purchasing (and rationing) an *in vitro* fertilisation service. *Br.J. Obstet. Gynaecol.*, **101**, 759–61
2. National Health Service and Community Care Act, 1990. (London: Her Majesty's Stationery Office)
3. National Health Service (General Medical Services Regulations) (1992) SI 1992 no.635. In Kennedy, I. and Grubb, A. (1994). *Medical Law.* (London: Butterworth)
4. NHS Act 1977. (London: Her Majesty's Stationery Office)
5. Redmayne, S. and Klein, R. (1993). Rationing in practice: the case of IVF. *Br. Med. J.*, **306**, 1521–4
6. Royal College of Obstetricians and Gynaecologists (1992). *Report on Fertility Treatments, Guidelines for Practice.* (London: RCOG Press)
7. *Effective Health Care* (1992). Number 3, School of Public Health, University of Leeds, Centre for Health Economics, University of York Research Unit, Royal College of Physicians
8. National Infertility Awareness Campaign (1995). *Reports of the Third and Fourth National Surveys of NHS Funding of Infertility Services.* (London: College of Health)
9. HFEA Annual Reports (1992, 1993, 1994 and 1995). (London: *Human Fertilisation and Embryology Authority*)
10. Loi no 94-653 du 29 Juillet 1994, relative au respect du corps humain et Loi no 94-654 du 29 Juillet 1994, relative au don, Assistance Médicale à la Procréation et diagnostic prénatal. (Paris: Journal Officiel du 30 Juillet 1994)
11. BMJ news (1997). Rationing is now accepted as inevitable by all sides. *Br. Med. J.*, **314**, 461
12. Smith, R. (1996). Being creative about rationing. *Br. Med. J.*, **312**, 391–2
13. Raphael, D. D. (1981). A theory of justice. In *Moral Philosophy*, p.71. (Oxford: Oxford University Press)

14. Winston, R. L. M. (1991). Resources for infertility treatment. *Baillières Clin. Obstet. Gynaecol.*, **5**, 551–73
15. Raphael, D. D. (1981). Intuitionism and objections to utilitarianism. In *Moral Philosophy*, p. 47. (Oxford: Oxford University Press)
16. Human Fertility and Embryology Act 1990. (London: Her Majesty's Stationery Office)
17. Dworkin, G. (1991). *Taking Rights Seriously*, p. 205. (London: Gerald Duckworth and Co. Ltd.)
18. Bromham, D. (1994). Should there be limits to IVF? Some public policy viewpoints. In *Ethics in Obstetrics and Gynaecology*, Ch.19. (London: RCOG Press)
19. Gillon (1994). The four principles plus scope. *Br. Med. J.*, **309**, 184–8
20. Benatar, S. (1996). What makes a just healthcare system. *Br. Med. J.*, **313**, 1567–8
21. Nisker, J. A. (1996). Rachel's ladder or how societal situation determines reproductive therapy. *Hum. Reprod.*, **11**, 1162–7

2

Ethics of embryo research

F. Shenfield and C. Sureau

INTRODUCTION

We attempt here an analysis of why it may be ethically or morally right or wrong to perform research on the human embryo. We are particularly concerned with the embryo *in vitro*, especially since the scientific and clinical landmark of the first human *in vitro* fertilization (IVF), resulting in a live pregnancy[1], has made the embryo available to the scrutiny of scientists outside the maternal environment.

Since then, one may ask whether and how the respect firmly articulated by Kant in his categorical imperative as owed to the person may be shown to the human embryo; and how we place research on this entity in the context of the child to be – a symbol of future generations towards whom we should be acting responsibly[2].

The term embryo has already given rise to a famous semantic debate: the use of the term pre-embryo, or 'the stage of the conceptus for the interval from the completion of the process of fertilization until the establishment of biologic individuation'[3], led to controversy, and suspicion that its human essence was deliberately being ignored or lessened by this prefix, branded as 'circumstantial ontology'[4].

It thus became clear that the status of the embryo must be qualified, if not defined. Academic lawyers have written essays on how this may fit into only two categories known by the law, i.e. 'res' (a 'thing') which can become property; or 'person', which cannot apply to the embryo[5]. A consensus seems to have emerged, on both sides of the Atlantic, opting for the term 'potential person'[6,7].

Thus, the human embryo deserves respect because of its 'potential' and kinship. Furthermore, this very notion of respect is enshrined in both the French legislation of 1994 (loi 94-653 concerns 'respect of the human body and its products'), and the British Human Fertilisation and Embryology Act (HUFE Act) 1990. The English Act set up the Human Fertilisation and Embryology Authority, whose *Code of Practice*[8] spells out that the respect of the embryo is 'fundamental to the Act', and delineates the duties and responsibilities of scientists and practitioners to their patients and the potential offspring this embryo may represent.

The practice of research on human beings has long been subjected to strict regulations. The purpose of this research must withstand scientific analysis, and be of a nature which is impossible to achieve in animal research. Consent to the research is the key to the respect of the autonomy of the subject concerned, and, in the case of the embryo, may be given by proxies, i.e. the male and female providers of the gametes at its origins.

Society in general has added its scrutiny to the detailed research undertaken under the microscope in the field of reproduction. This encompasses the specialist attention of philosophers, who state that the important question is 'when does life begin to matter morally?', rather than 'what is a person'[9]. Many debates on the subject have concentrated on the care and precautions to be taken in research, often defined by legal limits (French loi 94-654 of 1994, and British HUFE Act 1990), and the duty towards the future generation exemplified by the embryo and its human potential.

We first outline the ethical dilemmas raised by embryo research *per se* and argue for the inevitability of discussing, if not determining, its status and the necessity for research. We then analyze the implications of embryo research for diagnosis and therapy. In conclusion, we examine the possibility of reaching a consensus in Europe, and the duty one has to future generations to ensure safety of the applications of research.

THE NECESSITY FOR EMBRYO RESEARCH

Animal embryo research may not answer all the questions relative to the human embryo and its eventual ability to fulfil its potential. Not only does pathology often differ between species (for instance repeated miscarriage is specific to the human species), but the goals are often dissimilar, concentrating on 'quality' and commercial value in animals. An ethically acceptable goal in human medicine is the improvement of success rates in IVF. If IVF is morally acceptable, so is embryo research, the latter being necessary to improvement of the former. The position of the Catholic Church which forbids both, is just as logical. In this context, the end does not justify the means. At a recent meeting on the status of the embryo at the Council of Europe, however, it was stated that there was no objection to germinal therapy, provided the embryo was obtained by gamete intra-Fallopian transfer (GIFT) and lavage[10].

Advice and reflection are essential, but may only serve as guidelines at best. When society feels strongly enough about the matter concerned, legislation is enacted. Both the HUFE Act 1990 and the July 1994 loi reflect, in the UK and France, the intensity and breadth of public concern in matters of reproduction. Both laws avoid qualifying the status of the embryo as such, within the only two categories known in law: 'res' or 'person'. The HFEA *Code of Practice* stresses 'that the special status of the embryo is fundamental to the provisions of the Act' without defining this special quality, and the French law underlines the respect due to the human body 'as soon as life begins' without defining this precise moment.

It is also interesting to compare the English and French legislation, in which some research is allowed to rather different degrees, within specific boundaries and circumstances. The framework of the English legislation is dual: each research project has to be approved and granted a 3-year license by the HFEA, as long as it falls within five categories allowed in the Act: (1) promoting advances in the treatment of infertility; (2) increasing knowledge about the causes of congenital disease and (3) causes of miscarriage; (4) developing more effective techniques of contraception or (5) methods for detecting the presence of gene or chromosome abnormalities in embryos before implantation. Section 3 details the activities prohibited, amongst which are cloning, the creation of chimeras, trans-species transfer or the alteration of the embryonic genome. Finally, there is a time limit for *in vitro* research of 14 days or the appearance of the neural plate, for which the consensus is internationally far-reaching[11]. This does not so much reflect the principle of graduation and potentiality, as a compromise between varied interests, as in fact a 14-day embryo *in vitro* loses its potential to become human, and thus could arguably be experimented on more easily than a younger one[12].

The French legislation (loi 94-654) passed in July 1994 symbolizes the difficulty in finding a compromise that makes sense: it leaves a void of interpretation, stipulating that embryo 'experimentation' is forbidden, as is the conception *in vitro* of human embryos specifically for studies, research or experimentation. 'Studies' are allowed with a couple's consent 'in exceptional [undefined] circumstances' as long as they do not threaten the integrity of the embryo, and have the approval of the Commission Nationale de Médecine et de Biologie de la Reproduction et du Diagnostic Prénatal. As the term 'study' implies looking without touching (although pre-implantation diagnosis is allowed), and the difference between experimentation and research is not defined, it is not surprising that the *décrets d'application* are eagerly awaited. The task of the commission in this field is rather awe inspiring, and does not augur well for progress in view of the restrictive character of the legislation.

If one accepts that embryo research is permissible, two further problems arise: the source of embryos, and their fate. May one use non-viable embryos, the study of which may not lead to easily applicable results for viable embryos? May one use abandoned embryos, for which by definition there would not be the need for any consent to research, before they are due to be destroyed? In most cases embryos used for research will be destroyed, as the safety of the potential child who might ensue could not be assured, and it can actually be argued that it would be unethical to replace such an embryo *in utero*. Since the possibility of cryopreservation of embryos[13] has enabled couples to have further attempts at embryo transfer from one stimulatory IVF cycle, the creation of embryos purely for research purposes has been even more topical. French legislation makes this a criminal offence (Art 511-18), and the HUFE Act leaves to the HFEA the control of every single research project in the UK.

A *Convention on Bioethics* by the Steering Committee on Bioethics set up by the Council of Europe states that embryos may not be created with the intention of conducting research on them[14]. Three examples show the difficulty in applying this rule: (1) the study of cryopreservation of oocytes must be followed eventually by embryo formation to check on their normality; (2) if one manages to 'wash' HIV-positive semen and fertilize an oocyte, it would be unethical to replace the first embryo thus created; and (3) the studies of culture media with the aim of ensuring the lack of contamination with prions, for instance, will also necessitate the 'creation of embryos with the intention of conducting research on them'.

The same issue has given rise to a complex debate in the USA, after the report of the National Institutes of Health (NIH) Embryo Research panel had endorsed pre-implantation embryo research on the grounds that it offers potential benefits to infertile couples, and because the pre-embryo 'does not have the same moral status as infants or children'[15]. In the case of fertilization of embryos for research alone, the panel outlined two special categories according to the nature of the research of 'outstanding scientific and therapeutic value', including, for instance, research on freezing of oocytes followed by fertilization, or the comparison of embryos from couples 'at risk' of congenital defects and 'controls'. Within a few hours, a presidential statement directed the NIH not to support such research.

This dilemma about the source of the embryos can go one step further, with the theoretical possibility of using fetal material as a source of oocytes stemming from animal research, or ovarian graft[16]. In the UK, a public consultation by the HFEA on the matter of fetal sources, relating to both therapeutic use (when it would be technologically feasible), and research, was undertaken in 1994. Mostly for psychological reasons of unease, fetal material was deemed suitable for research, but not for therapeutic use[17].

Recently, the HFEA has allowed lengthening of the statutory limit for cryopreservation of embryos, which was initially 5 years from the application of the 1990 Statute, to 10 years from 1 May 1996. Nevertheless, one must contemplate the destruction of embryos whose gamete donors cannot be traced to lengthen their period of cryopreservation, and the *Code of Practice* recommends that it be done 'in a sensitive manner'[18].

THE CONSEQUENCES OF THE ACCEPTANCE OF EMBRYO RESEARCH

Once pre-implantation research on the embryo is accepted, it follows that the status of the embryo as a non-person is implicitly recognized. This is not because its consent cannot be obtained, as there are several instances in law where proxy consent is accepted (for children, or adults unable to give proper consent for reason of 'incapacity'); but rather because its destruction is necessarily planned, distancing the embryo more remotely from full human status. By definition, when the technique researched has been proven to be safe and useful, it may become therapeutic or diagnostic. Then the embryo concerned may be allowed to fulfil its potential to become a person – the legal person, which, in British law, it does not become until born alive (Congenital Disability (Civil Liability) Act 1975).

Cloning is another matter linked to research on pre-implantation embryos which has led to much debate. All types of cloning, namely nuclear transplantation, blastomere separation or bisection, elicit discomfort. Indeed blastomere separation gave rise to debate and strong statements ('if the aim of research is morally objectionable, all other ethical preconditions for research become irrelevant') in the pages of *Fertility and Sterility*[19].

The main objection to cloning, however, stems from the threat of trivializing the individual by replicating the entity 'embryo', with the consequence of creating identical potential persons: it would 'violate the inherent uniqueness and dignity of individuals' by deliberate twinning, if used to 'increase the number of embryos transferred, avoid subsequent egg retrieval, become a form of life insurance, or enable the selection of a desirable genome'[20].

Indeed, consent is one of the safeguards recognized internationally as an essential protection against the possible abuses stemming from embryo research[21].

CONCLUSION

In Europe and North America, consent represents one of the keys to consensus on the acceptability of pre-implantation embryo research. Consent of the gamete donors is the subject of the whole of Schedule 3 of the HUFE Act 1990, and is also enshrined in the French loi.

The other common principle, that of 'res extra commercio', is also stated in the HUFE Act 1990, with the exception of 'a sum as directed by the Code of Practice' for gamete donation. Its phasing out, planned in the HFEA *Annual Report*[22], would certainly increase the consistency of the principle stated (i.e. no money or benefit [to be exchanged] in respect of gametes and embryos) and strengthen the spirit of donation[23].

Amongst other safeguards, as in all research, openness is necessary, in order to enhance public participation in a debate which involves all members of society, not only the professionals concerned. This also means that all results should be published, that advice is sought from scientific and representative authorities on the French or British model, and that periodic reviews are planned to ensure updating of the legal constraints, if necessary. This is the case for the French loi which will be reviewed within 5 years.

The psychological aspects are intricate, and demand sensitive handling, which legislation may not perhaps always portray, although the opportunity for counselling is mandatory in English law (HUFE Act 1990).

In order to promote the understanding and tolerance of the advances of science, it is essential to give our patients better information on the rapid advances seen regularly in the field of reproduction, and their full implications. It is just as essential for the professional to listen to the concerns of potential patients and society at large, as we do not function in a vacuum.

It is very rare indeed that the aims of the two parties should not coincide: to fulfil our duty to the present and future generations. This raises the problem of the follow-up of children, without stigmatizing them by making them feel different from their peers. The past and present generations have seen changes in the legal age of voting, a symbol of the increased autonomy that society is willing to give its offspring. Discrepancies, as in the legal age of consent for sexual intercourse and consent to medical treatment (UK), or even between the legal voting age and drinking age (Sweden), epitomize the difficulties of such decisions at personal and societal levels. When is a child 'of mature understanding' (Gillick competent) to give continued consent (or dissent) to that to which his/her parents have consented on his/her behalf? This is going to be one of the most important ethical questions of the next century.

REFERENCES

1. Edwards, R. G., Steptoe, P. C. and Purdie, J. M. (1980). Establishing full term human pregnancies using cleaving embryos grown *in vitro*. *Br. J. Obstet. Gynaecol.*, **87**, 737–56
2. Fagot-Largeault, A. (1995). Procréation responsable. In Sureau, C. and Shenfield, F. (eds) *Ethical Aspects of Reproduction*. (Paris: John Libbey Eurotext)
3. Jones, H. W. and Schrader, C. (1989). And just what is a pre-embryo? *Fertil. Steril.*, **52**, 189–91
4. Sève, L. (1994). *Pour une critique de la raison bioéthique*. (Paris: Editions Odile Jacob)
5. Grubb, A. (1992). The legal status of the frozen human embryo. In *Challenges in Medical Care*, pp. 69–87. (London: J. Wiley)

6. Comité Consultatif National d'Ethique pour les Sciences de la vie et de la Santé (1984–1991). Avis concernant l'embryon, 1986 and 1990, avis relatif aux recherches sur les embryons humains *in vitro*, et sur les recherches soumises à un moratoire depuis 1986. Centre de documentation et d'information en ethique, INSERM 101 rue de Tolbiac, 75 654 Paris Cedex 13

7. Davis v. Davis (1992) 842 S.W.2d 605, Supreme Court of Tennessee. Reid, C. J., Anderson, Daughtrey, Drowota and O'Brien, J. J. In Kennedy, I. and Grubb, A. (eds.) (1993). *Frozen Embryos: Legal Status, Disposition and Control*, Davis v. Davis. *Medical Law Review*, Vol 1, Number 2, pp. 273–8

8. Human Fertilisation and Embryology Authority (1995). *Code of Practice.* (London: Human Fertilisation and Embryology Authority)

9. Harris, J. (1985). Beings, human beings and persons. In *The Value of Life*, pp. 10–18. (London: Routledge)

10. Bompiani, A. (1996). Aspects éthiques du diagnostic pré-implantatoire, troisième symposium sur la bioéthique, CDB 1/SPK (96) 11. (Strasbourg: Council of Europe)

11. FIGO Secretariat (1994). *The Study of Ethical Aspects of Human Reproduction.* (London: FIGO)

12. Baird, P. (1995). Research on pre-embryos (zygotes). In Sureau, C. and Shenfield, F. (eds) *Ethical Aspects of Human Reproduction.* (Paris: John Libbey Eurotext)

13. Trounson, A. and Mohr, L. (1983). Human pregnancy following cryopreservation, thawing and transfer of an 8-cell embryo. *Nature (London)*, **305**, 707–9

14. Council of Europe (1996). *Convention for the Protection of Human Rights and Dignity of the Human Being with Regard to the Application of Biology and Medicine: Bioethics Convention*, Strasbourg, November

15. Fletcher, J. C. (1995). US public policy on embryo research: two steps forward, one large step back. *Hum. Reprod.*, **10**, 875–1878

16. Gosden, R. G. (1990). Restitution of fertility in sterilised mice by transferring primordial ovarian follicles. *Hum. Reprod.*, **5**, 117–22

17. Human Fertilisation and Embryology Authority (1994). *Donated Ovarian Tissue in Embryo Research and Assisted Conception*, Public Consultation Document. (London: Human Fertilisation and Embryology Authority)

18. Shenfield, F., Matson, P. L., Hamer, F., Lieberman, B. A. and Steele, S. J. (1993). *The Statutory Limit for Embryo Storage in the U.K.: A Potential Problem for 1996.* (London: Centre of Medical Law Ethics)

19. Nisker, J. A. and Baylis, F. (1994). The best of us. Letter to the editor. *Fertil. Steril.*, **62**, 893–4

20. Robertson, J. A. (1994). *The Question of Human Cloning*, Report 24, No. 2 pp. 6–14. (New York: Briarcliff Manor)

21. American Fertility Society (1994). Ethical considerations of assisted reproductive technologies, by the Ethics Committee of the American Fertility Society. *Fertil. Steril.* (Suppl.), November

22. Human Fertilisation and Embryology Authority (1995). *Annual Report.* (London: Human Fertilisation and Embryology Authority)

23. Shenfield, F. and Steele, S. J. (1994). A gift is a gift is a gift or why gamete donors should not be paid. *Hum. Reprod.*, **10**, 253–5

3

Donating life: practical and ethical issues in gamete donation

G. M. Lockwood

INTRODUCTION

Although eggs and sperm have an equal genetic contribution to make to the production of an embryo and hence to a potential person, the difficulties attendant on obtaining donated eggs are so great (due to the novelty and complexity of the procedure and the low level of public awareness)[1], as compared to those surrounding donated sperm, that I shall concentrate in this paper mainly on eggs.

Acquiring sperm for donation is more straightforward – the university students who make up the majority of our donor pool refer jokingly to 'earning their beer money'. They are carefully screened and the selected and successful group (only a third of the initial volunteers) provide a high-quality product at low cost. The law ensures that no donor may father more than ten children (unless the donation is to provide a full sibling for an existing donor child). Donors are matched for height, skin, hair and eye color, blood group and sometimes religion, with the man who will be the *social* (and legal) father of any resulting baby. Although the parents of children born following the use of donor sperm are counselled and encouraged to tell their offspring of their origins, we know that the majority do not.

Why then should egg donation be perceived as so relatively problematic? In a society in which male primogeniture and inheritance are still the rule, it would appear that sperm and not eggs should lead to concern about gamete donation. The birth-mother is the legal mother under English Law whether or not she is the genetic mother, but issues of paternity have always been harder to determine and blood-group studies have found that in some areas above 5% of all children could not possibly be the genetic offspring of their putative fathers. By comparison, the number of children born as a result of gamete donation seems tiny and anxieties about the genetic identity of individual children seem misplaced. We have a situation of adequate supply of donor sperm, but for egg donation, the opposite is the case, with long waiting lists even in the commercial sector and desperate would-be recipients reduced to offering secret (illegal) inducements to egg donors.

The range of women who could benefit from egg donation is wide and growing wider, and advances in medical science (oncology and radiotherapy) and changes in life-style (delayed motherhood and 'designer babies') will maintain this growth. Women with spontaneous premature ovarian failure, or that induced by chemotherapy, radiotherapy or surgery, and those with maternally inherited genetic disease, recurrent miscarriage or repeatedly failed *in vitro* fertilization (IVF), all now recognize the role that donated eggs could play in helping them to achieve motherhood. And they are correct in this belief, since live-birth rates of over 50% after three cycles and 90% after five cycles of treatment are now routinely achieved in many IVF centers. Add to this group the older women who for career or other motives have chosen or been obliged to delay parenting until their chances of spontaneous and successful pregnancy are very low, and we see the origin of the current crisis of supply.

Male fertility has always extended decades beyond that enjoyed by women and the revolutionary new techniques in micromanipulation and assisted fertilization such as intracytoplasmic sperm injection (ICSI) have enabled men with extremely poor sperm function parameters to avoid recourse to donated gametes if they choose.

The Human Fertilisation and Embryology (HUFE) Act 1990 states clearly that 'No money or other kind of benefit shall be given or received in respect of any supply of gametes or embryos unless authorised by directions'. This has come to mean that £15 plus 'reasonable expenses' is payable. A directive of 1992 'allows the provision of treatment services and sterilisation in exchange for ovum donation'[2].

The overwhelming conviction underpinning this is clearly that the human body and its parts and products should remain *res extra commercium*, and public outrage in the UK about the sale of kidneys for donation which led to the 1989 Human Organ Transplant Act is readily reactivated at the prospect of paying egg donors for their eggs. I wish to argue that this anxiety, even outrage, is misguided and misplaced.

If we consider options for overcoming the shortage of egg donors in descending order of public perception of desirability, it appears that altruistic, unpaid, anonymous donors are considered to be the most desirable. Below these come *known* donors who are often related to the would-be recipient. After these come so-called 'introduced pool' donors who are recruited by a would-be recipient not for themselves but to speed their passage to the top of the waiting list for anonymous donors. Below these we have various 'egg-share' schemes. The most altruistic (and hence according to the conventional view the most ethically acceptable) is the woman undergoing IVF or gamete intrafallopian transfer (GIFT) who is responding well to ovarian stimulation and who is invited to consider giving up some of her eggs to another woman. This is most likely to occur when excellent fertilization rates for her own eggs are expected and when she does not wish to have spare embryos frozen. Slightly more ethically problematic are schemes in which subsidized or free IVF is offered to women who would not otherwise be able to afford IVF at all, in exchange for half their eggs[3].

A rung below this on the ladder of desirability are donors offered 'payment in kind', which in practice often means free laparoscopic sterilization at a private hospital, but the eggs may be 'cashed in' for other surgery such as varicose vein removal. I heard of one case in which the donor's son had free tattoo removal in exchange for his mother's eggs. 'Commercial' donors are almost universally disapproved of, since they are offered hard cash or high-cost consumer goods in exchange for undergoing stimulation and egg retrieval. Some sources of eggs are almost universally regarded as unacceptable, including aborted female fetuses and 'brain dead' road accident victims.

I wish to suggest that this 'ladder of ethical acceptability' should be completely inverted on the grounds not only that its philosophical premises are profoundly flawed, but also that its application serves greatly to diminish rather than to enhance the supply of eggs for donation.

EGG DONATION WITHOUT PAYMENT

To begin with altruistic donors, the 'gold standard' of donor morality, the problem is that there are simply not enough women prepared and able to make this commitment for free. However much a young mother (and the law says she must be under 36, and most authorities require, also, that she be multiparous, have completed her family, be using a fail-safe method of contraception and have the agreement and support of her partner, if any) may wish publicly to express her gratitude for the joy motherhood has brought her by helping a childless woman experience those unique pleasures, consider what she is letting herself in for. An uncomplicated egg-donation cycle will entail, including the treatment cycle visits, at least ten journeys to the fertility center if the legal requirements for counselling and screening are to be fulfilled. The woman will undergo hormonal manipulations involving the imposition of a temporary, and reversible, menopause followed by hyperstimulation and egg retrieval, with its attendant short-term risks of bleeding, infection and ovarian hyperstimulation syndrome (OHSS).

The long-term risks are not yet fully known but there is anxiety about the effects of fertility drugs on the female reproductive system[4-6]. As clinicians we should be prepared to question whether we should *allow*, let alone encourage, anyone to submit themselves to this in the name of altruism. Where altruistic anonymous donors are forthcoming, they frequently stipulate the type of woman for whom they are prepared to provide eggs[7]. In some surveys, 85% of donors have specified that they do not want their eggs to be given to 'old' women or single women. A recent survey of egg donation and ethnic minorities found that throughout the whole of the British Isles, only 17 women from ethnic minorities had volunteered to become anonymous egg donors in the past 2 years. This compares with 274 couples from ethnic minorities requesting egg donation in the same period[8].

The women who are prepared to become known donors are often sisters, cousins, neighbors or workmates of infertile women whose medical problems have resulted in sterility or whose fruitless quest for success with fertility treatments has rendered them objects of pity in the would-be donors' eyes. The hazards associated with egg donation are the same as for the altruistic donors, but in addition to this we have the problem of coercion. The would-be grandparents have been known to encourage donation between sisters, and where there is wide disparity of wealth between family members the opportunity for abuse is evident. I have experienced a situation in which an unmarried sister who already had four children conceived again just to avoid the unbearable family pressure to become an egg donor for her older sister with premature ovarian failure. This situation is also an encouragement to deceit. I was once confronted by two women whose claims to be sisters were disproved by blood tests; and it transpired that one was the wife of a former business partner of the other and that the planned 'donation' of eggs was in settlement of a large debt.

Even when coercion is not an issue, the relationship of the resulting child to a family member or close associate who is the genetic, but not the legal or 'birth' mother is fraught with potential difficulty. The inevitability of the outcome of the cycle being known means that in unsuccessful cycles there can be recrimination, and in successful cycles the egg donor may feel entitled to exercise unwarrantable interest in and control over the pregnancy and birth: 'I don't want *my* baby to have a Cesarean'. Minor disagreements on issues of child rearing and discipline can rapidly escalate in this atmosphere.

'Introduced pool' donor schemes, as described above, were heralded as a way to avoid the problem associated with the lack of anonymity between known donors. However, the altruism here is clearly stretched and the variability of the outcome, when known or even surmised, makes for great unhappiness. Imagine a situation in which the sister of a would-be recipient on a waiting list agrees to become a donor in 'the pool' so that her sister may be treated immediately. The altruistic sister unexpectedly overresponds to the gonadotropins and 20 good eggs are retrieved, but she is hospitalized with OHSS. Her sister's donor produces only two eggs, neither of which becomes fertilized. The sisters subsequently discover that all three of the women amongst whom the donor sister's eggs were shared conceived in that cycle and two even have frozen embryos in store! I contend that 'introduced pool' schemes may serve to draw attention to the plight of women needing donor eggs, but as far as individuals participating in the scheme are concerned, they may represent the worst of both worlds. The donors encounter all the risks associated with the treatment, but are only distantly and indirectly instrumental in the outcomes in which they are interested.

Altruistic egg-share schemes would seem to overcome many of the problems identified for the supposedly more desirable schemes discussed thus far. Women approached to share their 'excess' eggs are all good responders and likely, therefore, to do better than average with all types of artificial reproductive techniques (ART). However, they are by definition infertile and statistically less likely to conceive than the infertile recipients of their spare eggs. The relentless march of technology has to some extent brought about the demise of the altruistic egg-share scheme. This is because improved implantation rates for frozen embryos mean that the cost per baby born from frozen embryos already in store is lower than the cost of babies born from further fresh cycles, notwithstanding the reduced implantation rate of cryopreserved embryos. Even very young women requiring IVF are well aware that they are more likely to get a baby from one of their embryos made and frozen when they are 25 than from a fresh embryo made when they are 38. Again anonymity is theoretically guaranteed, but in small units it is possible for an 'unsuccessful' donor to discover, or just come to believe, that somebody else got a baby with one of *her* eggs.

Egg-share schemes in which donors receive free or subsidized treatment are apparently even more fraught with difficulties, for here donors may worry that the paying recipient(s) may be getting the better eggs! Subsidized donors who are themselves unsuccessful suffer either if the outcome is kept secret, in which case they do not know whether their eggs should be blamed for their continuing fertility problem, or if they are told that their recipient was successful, in which case the sense of injustice can be overwhelming. There is no getting away from the fact that women who give up half their eggs at IVF, because they could not otherwise afford the treatment at all, are doing so under pressure. But to prevent them from so doing, on the grounds that this represents unacceptable coercion, would surely be objectionably paternalistic. In Britain today, where only a tiny minority of IVF cycles are available on the National Health Service (NHS), and then to a highly restricted group of patients often after a long wait, we have a situation in which there are two groups of winners – poor women given access to IVF they otherwise could not afford and rich women receiving donated eggs they otherwise would not get – and no losers. This seems, on moral grounds, to be clearly preferable to any of the alternatives so far discussed.

EGG DONATION FOR PAYMENT

Egg donors who receive payment in the form of surgical or medical treatments unrelated to a fertility problem often have their motives questioned, but I feel they represent one of the morally worthiest groups of donors. The vast majority of such women are undergoing laparoscopic sterilization under general anesthetic, and therefore have already voluntarily embraced some of the most significant risks associated with being an egg donor. By definition they are all parous women who may feel some regret at some level for voluntarily relinquishing their fertility so absolutely and perceive that donating at the time of their sterilization allows some positive element to be retrieved from what is essentially a negative medical encounter. As a society we may value 'pure' altruism very highly, but we often feel more comfortable with the more subtle altruism such as that demonstrated by the woman who became an egg donor at the hospital that granted her a free (and successful) reversal of sterilization.

Commercial egg donation is almost universally the least well regarded – both by the public at large, who view it as almost on a par with prostitution, and by the medical profession, who claim that clinicians who advertise for paid donors (in the USA) are little better than pimps[9]. It has been argued that women will misrepresent their medical history if they would otherwise be disbarred from donating their eggs, and even that recipients would not want eggs from women whose sole motive for donating them was financial gain. These claims are clearly specious. The screening tests for would-be donors are very thorough (including compulsory testing for HIV before and after a 6 month incubation interval).

The majority of 'professional' donors in the UK are young women of *proven* fertility (unlike the majority of young student sperm donors), with children to support. They have no interest in the outcome of their donations other than the position it gives them on the unofficial league tables of donor success maintained by some agencies! They do not place limiting restrictions on the use to which their eggs may be put and they rarely have a partner whose need for counselling must be considered. Because they view their donation cycles as a form of, or alternative to, employment, they are far more flexible and punctilious about clinic visits than one-off altruistic donors who require a great deal of support and assistance. Most significantly, their receipt of a substantial sum of money in exchange for their eggs reflects a realistic recognition by themselves (and by the recipients) of the risks inherent in their donation cycle. I am aware of one such donor who was able to give up a life dependent on prostitution, and felt that the hazards of OHSS could not compare with those of life on the street. Another case was that of a young widow who was able to leave a low-paid job and stay at home with her children when her widow's pension was supplemented by three paid egg donation cycles a year.

CONCLUSION

In this paper, I have endeavored to show that commercial egg donation is far from being the morally dubious activity that it is often claimed to be, and in fact holds the key to the current severe shortage of donated eggs. By contrast, anonymous, unpaid, altruistic donation and known donation, whether direct or indirect, are revealed as limited and inherently limiting sources of eggs that carry significant risks, not only to the physical health of the donor (for which she gets little or no tangible compensation) but also to the psychological health of the donor, the recipient and, if the cycle is successful, to the child that is born. To use one group of infertile women to try to help another group of infertile women, as is the case with altruistic and compensated egg-sharing schemes, may seem to retain some appeal – if only to some vague sense of sisterly solidarity. But to exploit an artificial shortage in a way that simultaneously reduces the chances of one group (the poor donors who lose half their eggs) while making the other group (the rich recipients) use eggs of often unproven fertility is arguably to do both groups an injustice.

I alluded earlier to two 'unacceptable' sources of eggs – sources so far down the ladder of desirability as to be positively subterranean. Using eggs from aborted female fetuses (or, more probably, transplanting biopsies of fetal ovarian tissue containing primordial follicles) will soon be a practical possibility. However, the wave of public dismay and revulsion that greeted the announcement of this as a theoretical option was so strong as to preclude its application in the foreseeable future. Dame Jill Knight referred to the 'yuk factor' when describing her visceral response to the prospect of children being born whose genetic mothers had never existed. It may be irrational for a society that effectively condones abortion on demand to take this view, but it is vital that fertility research is perceived to be moving with public opinion rather than ahead of it. The same technology that permits the use of fetal tissue may soon allow us to biopsy and mature *in vivo* the unstimulated egg-containing tissue from adult volunteer donors who would face none of the hazards of a super-stimulated cycle.

The question as to whether the next-of-kin should be allowed to consent to a brain-dead relative becoming an egg donor in the same way that they can confer a gift of life by consenting to the removal of their relative's heart, lungs and kidneys does warrant consideration. The issue of an individual's consent is considered central to judgments about gamete donation, as demonstrated in the recent case of a widow refused permission to use her late husband's (perimortem aspirated) sperm to attempt to achieve a pregnancy, since his written consent had not been obtained. I suspect, however, that many people would wish to avoid even the theoretical possibility of grieving parents snatching at the prospect of 'perpetuating' a dead daughter through a 'grandchild' they would never know born as a result of the 'donation' of their daughter's eggs. The greatest danger inherent in the headlong rush to apply the rapid advances in the field of ART lies with the tendency for babies to be regarded as commodities. Far from encouraging this tendency, allowing egg donors to be paid a fee for their services would increase the supply of donor eggs and focus attention on the needs of a substantial and deserving group of infertile women.

REFERENCES

1. Bilijan, M. M., Taylor, C. T., Gosden, C. M., Jones, S. V., Malone, C. G. and Kingsland, C. R (1995). How acute is the shortage of oocyte donors in the UK? Results of a British national survey. *Br. J. Obstet. Gynaecol.*, **102**, 746–7
2. Human Fertilisation and Embryology Authority (1992). *Directions given under the HUFE Act 1990. Ref D 1991/2.* (London: Human Fertilisation and Embryology Authority)
3. Ahuja, K. K. and Simons, E. G. (1996). Anonymous egg donation and dignity. *Hum. Reprod.*, **11**, 1151–4
4. Fischel, S. and Jackson, P. (1989). Follicular stimulation in high tech pregnancies: are we playing it safe? *Br. Med. J.*, **299**, 309–11
5. Rossing, M. A. (1996). Ovarian cancer: a risk of fertility treatment? *J. Br. Fertil. Soc.*, **1**, 46–50
6. Bristoe, R. E. and Karlan, B. Y. (1996). The risk of ovarian cancer after treatment of infertility. *Curr. Opin. Obstet. Gynaecol.*, **8**, 32–7
7. Pennings, G. (1995). Should donors have the right to decide who receives their gametes? *Hum. Reprod.*, **10**, 2736–40
8. Birdsall, M. A. and Edwards, J. M. (1996). Demand for donated eggs by ethnic minority groups exceeds the supply. *Br. Med. J.*, **7065**, 1145
9. Sauer, M. V. (1996) Oocyte donation: reflections on past work and future directions. *Hum. Reprod.*, **11**, 1149–50

4

Surrogacy

V. English, A. Sommerville and P. R. Brinsden

INTRODUCTION

Surrogacy has been practiced, although rarely and clandestinely, since Biblical times. Recognition of its potential acceptability as a solution for infertility, however, came only recently. Like many aspects of reproductive medicine, surrogacy attracts controversy, although it probably happens most frequently without medical supervision. Within the UK, debate about surrogacy can be seen as a barometer of changing public attitudes and increasing toleration of 'unconventional' family arrangements. These changes in British public and professional opinion are not necessarily mirrored in other parts of Europe, however, where surrogacy is still frequently regarded as unacceptable. France, for example, prohibits surrogacy and officially views the practice as an inducement to child abandonment.

In Britain, too, in the mid-1980s, media and professional bodies reacted with horror to the admission of a British woman, Kim Cotton, that she had planned her pregnancy in order to relinquish the child for a lucrative financial settlement. This was condemned as 'baby selling'. Surrogacy was seen as a new twist in female exploitation; this time with other women as the oppressors. Career women, it was predicted, would simply pay or pressure others to bear their children. Babies would be commodities made to order in an increasingly consumerist society.

That the dire predictions have so far failed to materialize must in part be due to the fact that they grew from a lack of real understanding of the motivation of surrogates and of people who seek their services. No evidence has emerged to indicate that surrogacy occurs or is sought for trivial reasons of convenience. Thus, as public acceptance of various kinds of fertility treatment and awareness of the pain of involuntary childlessness have gradually developed, surrogacy appears to be cautiously recognized as a viable option of last resort. Changing attitudes are illustrated by parliamentary provision of 'parental orders' to regulate surrogate arrangements (see below), by increased medical involvement in the practice and by the first signs of consideration being given to the notion of publicly funded surrogacy[1].

Until recently surrogacy, like infertility itself, was kept secret but, as the stigmas diminish, health professionals are increasingly consulted about this option. Anecdotal evidence indicates that the incidence of surrogacy is increasing although no data are collected centrally. Because of the potentially complex medical, ethical, legal, emotional and psychological issues involved in surrogacy, however, it is unlikely ever to be used by more than a small minority.

Apart from adoption, 'natural' or 'partial' surrogacy was, until recently, the only means by which certain infertile women could have children. Partial surrogacy involves a woman agreeing to assist an infertile couple by allowing her eggs to be fertilized with the sperm of the male partner of the childless couple by insemination. Any child born to the surrogate mother is given to the 'commissioning couple' or 'intended parents', of whom only the male partner has supplied gametes. The advent of modern assisted conception techniques, including *in vitro* fertilization (IVF), permits the gametes of the intended parents to be used to create embryos *in vitro*. Transferred to the womb of the surrogate mother, who makes no genetic contribution, the fetus is gestated and relinquished at birth to the intended parents who are also the genetic parents of the child. This is termed 'IVF' or 'full' surrogacy.

INDICATIONS FOR TREATMENT BY SURROGACY

The principal medical indication for treatment of the intended parents using full surrogacy are cases in which the female partner suffers from congenital absence of the uterus or following hysterectomy for cancer or severe hemorrhage. Some women who have suffered repeated miscarriage and are thought to be incapable of carrying a child to term may also be suitable. Repeated failure of IVF treatment is a further indication. Medical conditions that make pregnancy life threatening, such as severe heart or kidney disease, may also be indications. In the UK patients are not considered for treatment by surrogacy purely for career or social reasons.

THE ROLE OF ETHICS COMMITTEES

In Britain, very few of the clinics providing assisted conception treatment also provide surrogacy. Most of these rely on local ethics committees for advice and support in the decision-making processes involved in this often controversial and ethically contentious treatment. At Bourn Hall Clinic, for example, where the first British IVF surrogacy treatments were carried out, the ethics committee has drawn up guidelines to assist the physicians and scientists providing the treatment. All full surrogacy arrangements, once they have been fully assessed by both the clinician and the counsel-lor, are taken before the independent ethics committee for discussion. Only if approval is given by the committee is treatment given. The com-mittee may approve or reject the arrangement, or refer it back to the clinician and counsellor for further review and information. Before agree-ing to any arrangement the committee will satisfy itself that attention has been paid, by all concerned, to the complex legal, ethical and practical considerations.

LEGAL CONSIDERATIONS

Parliament reacted swiftly in 1985 to the moral outcry raised by the Baby Cotton case, and passed the Surrogacy Arrangements Act. Hastily drafted, the Act prohibits commercial (but not voluntary) surrogacy agencies and outlaws advertising for or about surrogacy. It prevents anyone, other than the surrogate mother or intended parents, from acting on a commercial basis to initiate, negotiate or compile information to make a surrogacy arrangement. The activities of voluntary agencies, acting on a non-commercial basis, are outside its scope and remain unmonitored and unregulated. Contrary to popular belief, the Act does not prohibit pay-ments to surrogate mothers. It does, however, hamper them and their potential clients by prohibiting advertisements seeking or volunteering or offering to facilitate surrogacy services.

Five years later, the Surrogacy Arrangements Act was supplemented by the Human Fertilisation and Embryology (HUFE) Act 1990. This Act restricts what it terms 'licensable activities' to premises licensed by the statutory body, the Human Fertilisation and Embryology Authority (HFEA). Activities requiring a license include creating or using an embryo outside the body and using donated eggs, sperm or embryos. Treatments carried out by health professionals such as IVF or artificial insemination using donor sperm (which is the case in partial surrogacy, in which the surrogate mother is inseminated with sperm from the intended father) require a license and can only lawfully occur subject to HFEA monitoring.

The HUFE Act also clarified previous uncertainty about the legal status of surrogacy contracts by unambiguously declaring them unenforceable in law (s.36). Furthermore, it clarified legal parentage by defining the child's legal mother as the woman carrying it regardless of whether mother and child were genetically related (s.27). These two sections of the Act ensure that if the woman carrying the child changes her mind and keeps it, she is legally entitled to do so. If the woman or couple who originally wanted the child decide for some reason to reject it, the child remains the legal responsibility of the woman who bore it. The Act also defines the legal father, but this is more complex. Legal paternity, at birth, rests with:

(1) The surrogate mother's husband, if she is married;

(2) The partner of an unmarried surrogate mother, unless he can prove that he did not consent;

(3) The intended (commissioning) father, if the surrogate mother is without a partner and insemination occurred without medical help (i.e. self-insemination);

(4) Nobody, if the surrogate mother is partnerless and insemination occurred with medical help in HFEA licensed premises (HUFE Act 1990, s.28).

The fourth aspect of the HUFE Act relevant to surrogacy concerns 'parental orders' which are a legal mechanism for transferring parentage from the surrogate mother and legal father to the intended parents. Previously, the intended parents had to initiate standard adoption procedures, even when the child was genetically their own. Parental orders change that in cases where certain criteria are met:

(1) The child must be genetically related to one or both of the intended parents;

(2) The intended parents must be married to each other and both must be aged 18 or over;

(3) The legal (surrogate) mother and father must consent to the parental order;

(4) No money other than reasonable expenses can be paid in respect of the surrogacy arrangement unless payment has court authorization;

(5) At the time of the application, the child's home must be with the intended parents and one or both of them must be domiciled in the UK, Channel Islands or the Isle of Man (HUFE Act 1990, s.30).

Parental orders and adoption orders both transfer a child's legal parentage within a surrogacy arrangement but the original birth certificate remains. It can be accessed by the child at the age of 18 to discover the identity of the birth parents.

Challenges arising from developments in reproduction have been dealt with in the UK by the establishment of a statutory regulatory framework. By legislation clarifying the legal status of surrogacy contracts and legal parentage, it was hoped that potential disputes or exploitation of economically and socially vulnerable women could be avoided. Indeed, although hard evidence on all aspects of surrogacy is elusive, as far as can be judged from the continuing lack of major public controversy, it appears that the legislation and good practice guidelines[2] may have helped to avert some but not all the problems predicted when first the public confronted surrogacy. Some problems remain. Among them is the lack of regulatory or support mechanisms for voluntary agencies which can be established by anyone with an interest in so doing, regardless of their knowledge, skills or experience.

ETHICAL ISSUES IN SURROGACY

Despite the lack of evidence of continuing or grave problems associated with surrogacy, ethical concerns remain, not least because the practice has only relatively recently been conducted openly and therefore the full implications may only become evident with hindsight as the children, known to be born following a surrogacy arrangement, reach maturity and parenthood themselves. The pain and regret of failed agreements are clear, for example, in the very small number of cases in which the surrogate mother has decided to keep the genetic child of the intended parents. Arguments may arise between the surrogate mother and intended parents regarding the demarcation of their respective responsibilities. Alternatively, all of the adults involved may seek to dissociate themselves if a serious abnormality is detected during the pregnancy or the child is born seriously handicapped. Disputes may arise if prior to or during the pregnancy the intended parents attempt to impose restrictions on the surrogate mother's activities or habits which potentially affect the child's wellbeing, such as smoking or the use of alcohol or drugs. In brief, the potential psychological and emotional tensions for all the parties continue to be a subject of concern and speculation. On the basis of these concerns, it was initially argued that health professionals in Britain should have nothing to do with surrogacy and that children born in such arrangements should be taken into care. Such views now appear extreme but nevertheless the potential difficulties inherent in such arrangements should not be underestimated.

Health professionals may be involved with surrogacy in different ways and their ethical duties to each of the parties (child, intended parents, surrogate mother, existing children) will be determined largely by the extent of the involvement. Three levels of responsibility for health professionals have been identified:

(1) They may advise people considering self-insemination;

(2) They may be involved in generating the pregnancy; and

(3) They may provide antenatal care to an established pregnancy[2].

Arguably, the greater the involvement, the greater the ethical responsibility to ensure that foreseeable harm (to any party) is avoided. By this reasoning, health professionals who accept a duty of care for an already pregnant surrogate mother have less influence and arguably less ethical responsibility than those who agree to help in establishing the pregnancy. Health professionals informed that people intend to carry out self-insemination may not be able to influence the outcome apart from encouraging the parties to give careful consideration to the implications and ensure that they are aware of appropriate sources of advice, information, health testing and counselling. Given the psychological and other complexities which may arise, the duty to encourage awareness of counselling is of particular importance. Ethical obligations owed to any pregnant woman and her child are of the same order. Personal views, particularly negative views about the very concept of surrogacy, must not affect the quality of care and support provided. Indeed, more information or psychological support may be necessary.

It is widely recognized that where health workers help to establish a pregnancy using reproductive technology, they have a special ethical responsibility to ensure that the child will not be foreseeably disadvantaged. Although it is sometimes counter-argued that no duties can be owed to potential people who do not, and may never, exist, this view has been addressed by the HUFE Act (s.13(5)), which makes it clear that health professionals do have ethical responsibilities for children they help create. Those providing licensable activities have a legal obligation under the Act to consider the 'welfare of any child who may be born as a result of the treatment . . . and of any other child who may be affected by the birth'.

Such obligations are complicated in the case of surrogacy by the fact that either the surrogate mother and her partner, if she has one, or the intended parents could ultimately take on the role of social parents and thus enquiries must be made about the health and suitability of all parties. The HFEA's *Code of Practice*[3] recommends that where fertility treatment is requested, the treatment providers should bear in mind the following factors.

(1) The patients' commitment to having and bringing up a child or children;

(2) Their ability to provide a stable and supportive environment for any child produced as a result of treatment;

(3) Their medical histories and the medical histories of their families;

(4) Their ages and likely future ability to look after or provide for a child's needs;

(5) Their ability to meet the needs of any child or children who may be born as a result of treatment, including the implications of any possible multiple birth;

(6) Any risk of harm to the child or children who may be born, including the risk of inherited disorders, problems during pregnancy and of neglect or abuse; and

(7) The effect of a new baby on any existing child of the family.

The close involvement of other people in the way in which a woman or a couple approach conception, pregnancy and delivery can lead to conflict. The intended parents have a valid interest in how pregnancy and labor are managed when their hoped-for (and possibly their own genetic) child is involved. Ultimately, however, the woman experiencing the pregnancy and delivery must be able to conduct her life without undue interference and consent to or refuse what is done to her body.

Care of the various parties may be shared between more than one general practitioner, consultant, health team and health visitor. Alternatively, one doctor may be required to consider the interests of a range of people including the potential child, the surrogate mother, the intended parents and any existing children of either party. Balance must be maintained between the rights and needs of the various parties, with it borne in mind that, for example, the duty of confidentiality owed to each individual is not diminished by the fact that they have entered into an arrangement with others who have a legitimate interest in the outcome of the pregnancy. If, however, foreseeable serious harm may result, a breach of confidentiality, to an appropriate source, may be justified. Such cases may arise if, for example, individuals previously known to have abused or neglected children seek to participate in a surrogacy arrangement which may leave them with ultimate care and control of a child.

PRACTICAL ASPECTS OF TREATMENT BY FULL SURROGACY

In IVF surrogacy programs, intended parents wishing to be considered for IVF surrogacy are referred by their local consultant gynecologists or general practitioners. The couples are usually seen alone in the first instance and an in-depth consultation and counselling about the medical aspects of the treatment is carried out. They are told that the clinic is unable to provide assistance with finding a surrogate mother. Advice and counselling is given about this and they are informed of the various options, such as using a relative or friend as the surrogate mother, although particular care needs to be taken to avoid emotional pressure being brought on relatives or friends. Alternatively, a volunteer could be sought through a voluntary agency or patient support group.

When the intended parents have found a suitable surrogate mother, she and her partner are interviewed at length and a full explanation of the implications of acting as a surrogate mother is given to them. If she is thought to be suitable, then both the intended parents and the surrogate mother and her partner, if she has one, are counselled in depth by an independent counsellor. If the counselling process is also satisfactory and there is no other obvious reason that the arrangement should not proceed, most clinics will seek advice from their ethics committee before proceeding. In the program at Bourn Hall, for example, a report is prepared for discussion by the independent ethics committee and its final recommendations are always followed. It would generally be considered good practice to follow the recommendation of the ethics committee.

Management of the intended mother in full surrogacy

The intended mothers have usually been fully assessed by the referring consultant. Evidence of normal ovarian function is obtained by a history of cyclical premenstrual symptoms and often of symptoms of ovulation, and can be confirmed by checking the serum follicle stimulating hormone (FSH) and luteinizing hormone (LH) levels. The blood groups of the intended parents are requested in case the surrogate mother is Rhesus negative and both the intended parents are tested for hepatitis B (HBV), hepatitis C (HCV) and human immunodeficiency virus (HIV) status. Ovarian ultrasound scanning may also be carried out to confirm ovarian activity. Other investigations are carried out as necessary on an individual basis.

Following completion of the full medical assessment, counselling process and approval by the ethics committee, treatment of the intended parents is started only when the surrogate mother has been identified and also fully counselled and approved by the ethics committee. Since most of the women requesting full surrogacy have entirely normal ovarian function, the management of their treatment cycles is as for normal IVF. With IVF surrogacy all embryos are frozen for 6 months 'quarantining' for HIV prior to uterine transfer to the surrogate mother, unless the sperm has previously been frozen for 6 months. This quarantining process is required, since the sperm of the male partner, in surrogacy, is considered under the same regulations as donor sperm.

Management of the surrogate mother

Surrogate mothers must be medically normal fit women, usually less than 37 years of age who have had at least one child. In the UK it is widely accepted that she should be married or in a stable heterosexual relationship and her husband or partner must be made fully aware of the implications of what his partner is doing in acting as a surrogate mother. Fertility investigations are not necessary. All surrogates and their partners are tested for HBV, HCV and HIV status. Before embryo transfer is carried out the HIV status of the intended parents is tested again.

If the surrogate mother is taking the oral contraceptive pill then it is discontinued one or two cycles before the replacement cycle and barrier methods of contraception are recommended. Strong emphasis is placed upon the need for reliable contraception. Embryo transfer is carried out either in a natural cycle without the use of any hormone treatment, or in a hormone-controlled cycle. A hormone-controlled cycle is recommended if the menstrual cycles of the surrogate are irregular, if she is found not to be ovulating regularly or if luteal phase insufficiency is suspected.

Results of treatment

The results of treatment by IVF surrogacy at Bourn Hall Clinic over the past 4 years are summarized here, to give an idea of the sort of chances of success that couples might be expected to achieve with this treatment: 27 intended parents undertook 44 IVF stimulation cycles and produced a mean of 9.6 (range 2–24) oocytes and 4.7 (range 1–13) embryos for freezing. A mean number of 2.1 frozen/thawed embryos were subsequently transferred to 30 surrogate mothers in 40 embryo transfer cycles. A clinical pregnancy rate of 42.5% (17/40) per transfer, 56.7% (17/30) per surrogate and 55.5% (15/27) per intended parent couple was achieved. The 'delivered baby rate' per surrogate was 41.4% (12/29) and per intended parent couple 44.4% (12/27).

The relatively high pregnancy and delivery rates are attributable to the fact that embryos from young women are placed in the uterus of young and normally fertile women.

CONCLUSION

In Britain, full surrogacy is now an accepted method of treatment for women who, for a number of reasons, are unable to carry their own child. It is only available in a very few specialist clinics and will only ever be an appropriate treatment option for a small number of women. Full surrogacy is a demanding process, both physically and emotionally. It involves a full medical assessment in a specialist IVF center, in-depth counselling and legal advice, followed by ovarian stimulation, oocyte collection, fertilization with the partner's sperm and the subsequent transfer of up to three embryos to the uterus of the surrogate mother. Partial surrogacy, involving insemination of the surrogate mother with the intended father's sperm is physically less demanding and less time-consuming, but does not allow both the intended parents to contribute to the genetic make-up of the child. Both partial and full surrogacy bear the same legal, ethical and emotional complexities which need to be carefully considered and understood.

The regulatory framework and good practice guidelines established in Britain attempt to encourage openness and informed decision-making and, arguably, have increased awareness and minimized the possibility of problems and abuse. The very profound issues raised by surrogacy, combined with the potential for complications, disappointment and exploitation, however, mean that it remains a controversial treatment and one on which European consensus has not been, and is unlikely to be, forthcoming. A useful comparison can be drawn between the approach taken to surrogacy in the UK and that taken by France, both seeking to protect vulnerable groups and uphold good ethical practice. Whether this objective is best achieved by prohibition, as in France, or by regulation, as in the UK, remains to be seen.

REFERENCES

1. (1996). Surrogate birth to be carried out on the NHS. *The Independent*, 13 January
2. British Medical Association (1996). *Changing Conceptions of Motherhood. The Practice of Surrogacy in Britain.* (London: British Medical Association)
3. Human Fertilisation and Embryology Authority (1995). *Code of Practice,* para 3.17 (London: Human Fertilisation and Embryology Authority)

5

The ethics of sex selection

J. A. Nisker and M. Jones

This exploration begins with a journey: a journey to understand the space occupied by women impelled to sex determination, a journey to the space occupied by physicians offering this service, a journey to a place we cannot go. But on a gray November evening in 1996, we shared the surface of the road taken by many South Asian women, travelled by four that very evening, from their south Vancouver Canada homes across the border to the gray strip-mall building in Blaine, USA, leased to Koala Labs.

Blaine is a town birthed by cross-border shopping. Its stores boomed until the sinking of the Canadian dollar subverted their existence. But cross-border shopping continues for some commodities and services. Dr John Stephens opens his Koala Labs clinic two evenings a month. He offered permission for our journey, just as he offered permission through Canadian newspapers for the journey of Canadian women to sex determination.

In Canada, a woman has government-funded access to ultrasonography for the purposes of fetal health, but not for sex predetermination. Abortion is also government funded, but abortion for sex selection is condemned (Canadian Medical Association[1], and Society of Obstetricians and Gynecologists of Canada[2]) and may soon be illegal (Human Reproductive and Genetic Technologies Act). Canadians interested in fetal sex selection must travel to the United States for sex determination; if a female is identified, they may have the termination in Canada, as long as the true reason remains unknown to the Canadian physician.

Science does not operate in a vacuum; context influences how a technology is used. The stories of women journeying to Koala Labs emerge from a tableau of conflict: cultural conflict, conflict within the practice of medicine, and disparate political positions translated from national and institutional health care visions. This chapter overviews the cultural context as well as the arguments for and against medical embrace of sex selection.

CULTURAL CONTEXT

Dr Stephens comes to the attention of Canadian couples by advertising the services offered in his clinic in the Vancouver Indo-Canadian newspaper, printed in Punjabi[3,4]. In our interview he described his patients as 'all Asians, the majority Southeast Asians of Sikh origin, and occasionally Muslims, Chinese and Koreans'. Indeed, despite the worldwide nature of male preference, the practice of the use of sex selection technology is focused on Asian cultures but the journey to Blaine for most women originally started in India. Along with China, Indian use of sex selection is the highest in the world. Both countries have sex ratio imbalances in regions where the practice is most prevalent[5]. Advocates of social justice in these countries have accomplished legislative change but continue to struggle against cultural codes that devalue women and condone this and other misogynist practices.

Kusum[6] feels the dowry system is the greatest cause for femicidal practices in India. At birth, a baby girl is seen as a liability: her living expenses will be carried by her parents until she marries, at which point she will not only abandon them, but take with her the resources accumulated in her dowry. Male children, conversely, bring wives and their dowries into the home to help support their parents through old age[6-8]. Male sex selection is obviously not a matter of a vast number of women preferring male children, or even being coerced into aborting by family members; rather it is part of a woman's socialization that babies of her own sex are not wanted. It would appear that devaluation of daughters, abortion of potential daughters, or commission of female infanticide may not always be against the woman's will; she may truly believe that it is the appropriate path to follow.

In a 1992 study conducted by the Community Services Guild of Madras of 1250 rural families, 249 families admitted to commission of female infanticide. Of these, 111 had done so in the 2 years preceding the study[6]. Indian social activists have lobbied for years to institute changes, and have met with some success. Although the Dowry Prohibition Act was brought into effect in 1961[9], this has failed to obliterate the practice. In January 1996, the 1994 Pre-Natal Diagnostic Techniques (Regulation and Prevention of Misuse) Act outlawing prenatal testing for the purposes of sex determination was finally effected[8]. The Act outlines punitive fines and imprisonment for encouragement of sex determination tests by relatives, advertising by clinics and revelation of fetal sex by ultrasonography unless for specific medical reasons. Practitioners who violate this law may permanently lose their license. The success of this legislation remains to be seen. As long-term changes cannot be effected without travel to the heart of the culture, there is concern that sex determination and selection will continue underground[8].

In the 'western ethic', a conflict occurs in attempting to negotiate cultural sensitivity (in the interest of human rights) and prevention of violence against women (also in the interest of human rights). Canada boasts a cultural mosaic, but its achievement is complex. We encourage the philosophy that when an individual leaves their country, they need not leave their culture behind. We strive for all cultures to achieve respect and be valued as contributing to our society. Yet just as Canadian culture cannot pretend innocence of human rights abuse in its historical development, it must recognize that the continuity of cultural beliefs of modern immigrants may conflict with the adopted culture, which diminishes both cultures by reinforcing harmful stereotypes. South Asian, as all cultures, prefer to struggle within to change practices that have been harmful to their populace, and hesitate to accept Western interference in this process.

We cannot presume to speak for immigrant women. But we can recognize that, although each individual has unique experiences, immigrant women share a set of situational characteristics that obstruct their achievement of maximally informed choice. Immigrant women enter a society often unfamiliar, and are encouraged to adopt different cultural norms, often in a different language, leaving their support networks behind. Although they may enter a new support network of immigrants when they arrive[10], women entering Canada from cultures more female-devaluing may perpetuate these attitudes. Culture follows immigrants not only in ceremonies, costumes and folk songs, but also in an internalized way of perceiving environment and interactions.

Socioeconomic factors can have a considerable impact on treatment options. Worldwide, the decision-making power of women seeking reproductive care is diminished when they are financially disadvantaged[11]. Poor employment avenues and the financial stresses of starting a new life may force some immigrant families to live in outright poverty. As Pilowsky states, 'poor women have less power than other women to make decisions regarding their health'[10]. Perhaps worst of all, those coming from a women-oppressive culture may be suffering from this oppression within their own home – from their male partners, female figures and from themselves. As a group, therefore, immigrant women's risk of being victimized by the use of medical technologies is magnified.

ARGUMENTS FOR SEX SELECTION

In the past several years, social justice concerns have encouraged cultural sensitivity as a human rights issue. Western cultures have often assumed the stance of moral superiority, acting as a role model for cultures that are, it is implied, 'backward'. It may be argued that preventing a woman from accessing sex determination of her fetus is a culturally imperialistic move that denies the woman respect for her rights.

At the International Federation of Gynecology and Obstetrics (FIGO) *International Symposium on Ethics in Reproductive Medicine and Biology*, the most commonly voiced reservation regarding a ban on sex selection abortion was that changes must originate in the culture rather than be forced upon a culture, or legislation might harm those it intends to protect[12]. If the culturally encrypted status of women is not addressed, the bearers of these children will be punished for their motherhood, and girls may live lives of poor quality or abuse and neglect. Furthermore, women from cultures in which sons are valued much higher than daughters may continue to have child after child until a son is achieved, creating huge families of undervalued women. Where family size is legislated, such as China, or economically restricted, an increase in infanticide may result.

Dr Stephens consistently defends 'gender identification' as beneficial for women culturally entwined, part of protection of all women's right to choose, part of the independence of patient and physician to comply with society's legal limit. Dr Stephens further argues that the technology he uses is, in itself, amoral, as he performs only sex determination, a process independent of sex selection. He also argues that more terminations would occur without sex determination's guarantee of males in half the cases. Some opponents to sex selection argue that, without the potential for ultrasonographic sex identification, families unwilling to accept a female fetus could use contraceptive strategies, but the couples accessing Dr Stephens' services are not only reluctant to have daughters, but strongly motivated to have sons. As only female pregnancies are undesirable, the motivation for male children negates the argument that couples unable to select the sex could turn to contraceptive strategies.

The argument Dr Stephens returns to is patient autonomy. He defends his work as ethically sound, on the basis of protecting the patient's right to receive the health care she seeks. He agrees with Hook[13], who states:

> ... [if] the patient was willing to pay for prenatal diagnosis that would result in information that was so-called non-medical, such as sex information as a by-product of the procedure, that the patient should still have access to that procedure and have access to that information, and there should be no coercion or withholding of information by the physician ...

Dr Stephens states:

> What I've essentially done is eliminated the authoritativeness, paternalism, patriarchy of physicians, physicians' power, and enhanced the autonomy of the patient in decision-making and taking responsibility.

Dr Stephens feels that it is every couple's right to know the sex of their baby. He feels the best care is that which respects the patient's right to make their own decisions.

ARGUMENTS AGAINST SEX SELECTION

The cultural encoding that enables sex selection does not exist unquestioned; indeed, the greatest criticism of sex selection abortion comes from South Asia and South Asian immigrant communities. Legislation prohibiting sex selection in India is among the strongest in the world. Shashi Asanand, Executive Director of the Vancouver Multicultural Family Support Services, is outspoken in her claim that women of South Asian origin remain pawns in a centuries-old society-induced quest for male children. She is concerned that many Canadian couples of South Asian origin continue to feel that a male child is required to validate their marriage, and thus comply with sex selection[14]. Sunera Thobani, former President of the National Action Committee of the Women of Canada, is of Sikh origin. Thobani is concerned that Koala Labs' advertising gives: 'the implicit notion...that South Asian culture celebrates and condones this particular form of misogyny'[4]. She goes on to assert that not only does Dr Stephens' marketing focus on South Asians serve to fan the flames of racial hostility, but it also obscures the global nature of the sex selection problem[4].

Collateral evolution of medical technology may abrogate its original motivation to improve human life. Ultrasound was originally developed to avoid potentially harmful X-ray exposure to the fetus during fetal age assessment, fetal head and pelvic wall measurement and placental localization. The determination of fetal sex was an incidental consequence of fetal age assessment at 10–12 weeks (through male genital visualization). Therefore, in a discussion of sex selection, the factors that influence decisions to use these technologies in this manner must be considered. As the Canadian philosopher Susan Sherwin suggests, those who control access to the technology are not those who are most in need of it. She warns of a 'professional elite' making decisions reflecting culturally constructed social biases that are 'sexist, homophobic, racist, capitalist, and elitist'[15]. The very act of targeted marketing in the manner Dr Stephens chooses lends credibility to the practice, as he is in a position of perceived authority. Morgan states that all women are subject to devaluation and infantilization at the hands of 'experts' in decisions involving medical technologies[16]. Raymond refers to male sex selection as the 'previctimization of women'[16]. Although activists in India and abroad are working to change the traditional perceptions that devalue women, western policies continue to foster and accommodate preference for male babies. Sherwin considers that women should be given the power to fight the coercion and refuse the use of the technology[15].

In their submission to the Canadian Royal Commission on New Reproductive Technologies, Immigrant and Visible Minority Women of British Columbia, along with similar groups, strongly stated their opposition to the effect that sex selection targeting has on a community long struggling against the devaluation of women[17]. Similar situations of 'market infiltration' have been noted elsewhere in Canada, most notably taking advantage of the large Asian community in Toronto and its proximity to New York State[3].

Proposed Canadian legislation barring sex selection cites serious risks to human health and safety, the dehumanization of motherhood, diminished value of human individuality and violation of the principle of non-commercialization of reproduction. Although the proposed Canadian Human Reproductive and Genetic Technologies Act would make sex selection abortion illegal, it may not decrease the number performed in Canada, as sex determination will remain available in the United States and depression, rather than an unwanted female fetus, would be the likely reason given to the consulted gynecologist. Indeed, depression is real for women torn between the desire to continue a pregnancy and pressures from culture and community.

In a 1991 survey of health professionals encountering abortion, Evans and colleagues[18] concluded: 'Abortion for sex selection violates equality in a radical way. Also, sex is not a disease, and to abort for sex is a precedent to eugenics.' These American authors feel limits should be placed on those 'assisting with abortions or selective terminations'[18]. Although Western cultures may remain patriarchal, most condemn as misogyny such deliberate femicidal practices as sex selection abortion.

INTERNATIONAL AND NATIONAL PROFESSIONAL ORGANIZATIONS

Professional associations are now issuing statements on sex selection. FIGO issued a position on sex selection in 1994. While its Committee for the Study of Ethical Aspects of Human Reproduction recognized 'that the ethical principle of protection of the vulnerable and the ethical principle of justice are violated by sex selection abortion (whether male or female)', it qualified that 'the ethical principle of autonomy of the woman would be violated by complete prohibition of sex selection abortion'. They believed that preconceptional sex selection was justifiable in the case of sex-linked genetic disorders and possibly for family balance, yet they warned that it 'should never be used as a tool for sex discrimination against either sex, particularly female'[12].

Of the participants in the debate, all agreed that in theory sex selection was abominable, and most agreed that it should be outlawed. Although the FIGO Ethics Committee condemned the practice, the members felt that they could not take the choice to terminate a pregnancy away from the woman who is pregnant. Another participant cautioned that doctors should not be making decisions regarding the use of reproductive technologies alone; society must guide them[12].

In 1994, the Commonwealth Medical Association stressed opposition to the use of the practice for discriminatory purposes:

> Physicians must never acquiesce in the wrongful use of sex selection procedures for purposes of discrimination. Whilst gender selection may be acceptable for the purpose of avoiding the transmission of genetic disease, it should be employed only selectively and sparingly for this purpose, and its use for sex discrimination must be condemned.[19]

The Canadian Medical Association's position on sex selection states that:

> Techniques of artificial sex selection for non-medical reasons should be prohibited as being contrary to the principle of equality of persons . . . [the Association] rejects the notion that one sex is inherently preferable to or better than another.[1]

The Society of Obstetricians and Gynaecologists of Canada issued a policy statement in 1994 that medical technologies are appropriately used to detect and minimize genetic diseases, but their use to support a societal discrimination against one sex in favor of another should be condemned:

> Measures designed to support societal preferences for male children whether by selective implantation of embryos, selective abortion of healthy fetuses after amniocentesis or infanticide, all reinforce discriminatory attitudes towards women and female children. Any similar attempt to favor birth of female children would be discriminatory against males.[2]

The American Society for Reproductive Medicine released the report of their Ethics Committee in 1994[20]. Although no chapter was devoted solely to sex selection, some consideration was given to the issue in their discussion of preimplantation genetic diagnosis. After a discussion of the value of preimplantation genetic diagnosis in identifying X-linked disorders, the committee stated that the use of preimplantation genetic diagnosis *solely* for sex selection was not acceptable; however, in its recommendations, it qualified that statement:

> The Committee finds highly problematic the use of gender selection to achieve 'family balancing' or other preferential goals based on nondisease traits. However, it may be premature to declare that there are absolutely no circumstances under which gender selection should be used, regardless of the technology involved in achieving it.

PRECONCEPTION AND PREIMPLANTATION SEX SELECTION

Sex selection can be attempted prior to fertilization by sperm sorting (still far from accurate), or preimplantation genetic diagnosis during the *in vitro* fertilization process (returning only embryos of the desired sex to the womb). There may be different degrees of moral acceptance of non-abortion methodologies. For example, from an antiabortion standpoint, sperm sorting would be the least objectionable method, since it occurs pre-fertilization, or pre-life. For those who are pro-life but feel that life does not begin until an embryo is implanted in the womb, then the IVF method may not pose a dilemma. For those who feel that the misogyny is the overriding problem, these methods of sex selection may be equally culpable to sex selection abortion.

At the FIGO conference[12], the following question was asked: 'As technologies become more accessible, e.g. preconception sex selection kits available at the drugstore, how can they be monitored?'. As stated above, FIGO's statement on preconception sex selection noted the complexity of the issue, especially regarding autonomy vs. protection of the vulnerable, but asserted that sex selection should never be employed for sex discrimination. However, FIGO's position on preconception sex selection differs from its position on sex selection abortion. It states:

> Preconceptional sex selection can be justified on social grounds in certain cases for the objective of allowing children of the two sexes to enjoy the love and care of parents. For this social indication to be justified, it must not conflict with other society values where it is practiced.

Do all cases of sex selection send the message that life of a certain sex is more valuable than life of another? Internationally, children of the male sex are preferred[8,21]. Even in cases in which sex selection is used for 'family completion' or 'family balance', there is a marked trend for families to select a male child as firstborn, which arguably has negative consequences for females[8,21]. Do all sex selection techniques perpetuate the existence of women as second-class citizens?

CONCLUSION

Stephens listened to our concerns about potential coercive influences in a woman's decision to attend his clinic, about the negative message regarding female worth, and about the cross-border shopping complexity that makes Canadian physicians and indeed our healthcare system complicit by performing sex selection abortion in Canada. His main retort – that the choice of whether or not to continue a pregnancy is in many societies considered an essential freedom for women – is unfortunately in the case of sex selection a misuse of the word 'choice'. However, on leaving Koala Labs, where patients' autonomy rather than misogynist practice was honestly argued, we could no sooner condemn Dr Stephens than condemn the couples in his waiting room. We can condemn the cultural impulse complicit with this moral misdirection, be it South Asian, American or Canadian, and search for resolution. Are sociocultural problems compelling women to seek sex determination by ultrasound and ultimately sex selection abortion assuaged by the existence of this technology, or reinforced? Should Dr Stephens and other ultrasonographers restrict their services to couples carrying genetic disease? Should women be questioned as to the motivation for requesting sex determination? Can Dr Stephens and other physicians who offer sex determination truly disconnect sex determination from the ultimate result of the information gained? It is hard to argue against all knowledge having worth, but if sex determination by ultrasound was not available, sex selection abortion would not occur. Regardless of the personal or cultural motivation, the message that sex selection for non-medical reasons sends to broader society is the suboptimal worth of women and thus of all human life.

REFERENCES

1. Canadian Medical Association (1994). *Position on sex selection*
2. Society of Obstetricians and Gynecologists of Canada (1994). http://sogc.medical.org/sogc_docs/public/guidelines/gender.htm. February 1, 1997
3. Thobani, S. (1992). Making the links: South Asian women struggle for reproductive rights. *Can. Woman Stud.*, **13**, 19–22
4. Thobani, S. (1993). From reproduction to mal[e] production: women and sex selection technology. In Basen, G., Eichler, M. and Lippman, A. (eds.) *Misconceptions*, pp. 138–54. (Hull, Quebec: Voyageur)
5. (1991). Facts on file. *World News Digest*, May 23, p. 186D1
6. Kusum, K. (1993). The use of pre-natal diagnostic techniques for sex selection: the Indian scene. *Bioethics*, **7**, 149–65.
7. Ward Anderson, J. and Moore, M. (1993). The burden of womanhood: Third world, second class. *Washington Post*, April 25
8. Rajan, V. G. J. (1996). Will India's ban on prenatal sex determination slow abortion of girls? *Hinduism Today*, **18**. http://www.HinduismToday.kauai.hi.us/ashram/April 96.html#gen241. February 1, 1997.
9. (1988). Facts on file. *World News Digest*, Dec. 16, p. 930D2
10. Pilowsky, J. E. (1991). A population at risk. *Healthsharing*, **12**, 21–4
11. Nisker, J. A. (1996). Rachel's ladder or how societal situation determines reproductive therapy. *Hum. Reprod.*, **11**, 1162–7
12. Sureau, C. and Shenfield, F. (1995). *Ethical Aspects of Human Reproduction.* (Paris: John Libbey Eurotext)
13. Hook, E. B. (1994). Prenatal sex selection and autonomous reproductive decision (letter). *Lancet*, **323**, 55–6
14. Asanand, S. (1996). Personal communication

15. Sherwin, S. (1989). Feminist ethics and new reproductive technologies. In Overall, C. (ed.) *The Future of Human Reproduction.* (Toronto: The Women's Press)
16. Morgan, K. P. (1989). Of woman born? How old-fashioned! – New reproductive technologies and women's oppression. In Overall, C. (ed.) *The Future of Human Reproduction.* (Toronto: The Women's Press)
17. Baird, P. (1993). *Proceed with Care: Final Report of the Royal Commission on New Reproductive Technologies.* (Ottawa: Canada Communications Group)
18. Evans, M., Drugan, A., Bottoms, S. F., Platt, L. D., Rodeck, C. A., Hansmann, M. and Fletcher, J. C. (1991). Attitudes on the ethics of abortion, sex selection, and selective pregnancy termination among health care professionals, ethicists, and clergy likely to encounter such situations. *Am. J. Obstet. Gynecol.*, **164**, 1092–9
19. Commonwealth Medical Association (1994). *Medical ethics and human rights: guiding principles.* (London: British Medical Association)
20. American Society of Reproductive Medicine (1994). Preimplantation genetic diagnosis. *Fertil. Steril.*, **62** (Suppl. 1), 64–6S
21. Katz Rothman, B. (1987). *The Tentative Pregnancy: Prenatal Diagnosis and the Future of Motherhood.* (New York: Penguin Books)

6

Ethical considerations of intracytoplasmic sperm injection

A. Van Steirteghem, H. Tournaye, C. Sureau and F. Shenfield

BACKGROUND

Until recently, the use of conventional *in vitro* fertilization (IVF) for patients with male factor infertility had indicated that a number of couples could not be helped since no or almost no fertilization occurred in patients with severely impaired semen. It was obvious that certain couples could not be accepted for IVF since too few spermatozoa with normal motility and morphology were present in the ejaculate; this, of course, includes patients with obstructive and non-obstructive azoospermia. The use of donor sperm was the only means by which to have children for most men with extremely altered semen parameters or azoospermia. Several forms of assisted fertilization, such as partial zona dissection or subzonal insemination, were occasionally reported to produce fertilization and births.

In 1992, the Brussels Free University Center for Reproductive Medicine reported the first pregnancies and births after a novel procedure of assisted fertilization, in other words intracytoplasmic sperm injection (ICSI), the direct injection of a single spermatozoon into the cytoplasm of the oocyte by means of micromanipulation[1]. It soon became clear that ICSI gave much better and more consistent results than other assisted fertilization procedures[2]. Today, ICSI can be carried out successfully with ejaculated, epididymal and testicular spermatozoa. ICSI has become the first-choice assisted reproductive technology to treat male infertility and within 5 years this technique has become available throughout the world.

A subpopulation of patients is known to have a higher incidence of genetic traits causing the infertility problems[3,4]. A major concern is related to the presence of microdeletions on the long arm of the Y chromosome. These deletions may be associated with testicular dysfunction, leading to extreme oligozoospermia or azoospermia. Using ICSI, such Yq microdeletions may be transmitted to the male offspring. Candidate fathers can be screened for these deletions; however, most of them are *de novo* deletions arising in the germinal cell line and thus routine screening is of limited value. Fathers with Yq microdeletions should be counselled that eventually they will transmit a microdeletion to their sons.

Another concern is gene mutations and deletions related to male subfertility and infertility. Most azoospermic patients with congenital bilateral absence of the vas deferens (CBAVD) have deletions or mutations of the cystic fibrosis gene. CBAVD can be considered as the genital form of cystic fibrosis. For this reasons, all CBAVD patients and their female partners should be screened for these deletions before starting any ICSI treatment with epididymal or testicular spermatozoa. If the female partner is a carrier of gene deletions or mutations, preimplantation or prenatal diagnosis should be proposed because of the risk of having a child with cystic fibrosis[5].

In patients with extreme oligoazoospermia, a substantial proportion of spermatozoa may be disomic or nullisomic. Prenatal karyotyping of ICSI offspring has shown that the incidence of sex chromosome aneuploidy is slightly elevated, i.e. around 1.0% instead of 0.2–0.3% in a large series of prenatal karyotypes after chorionic villus sampling. This increased incidence of sex chromosome aneuploidy in ICSI offspring can be explained more by this higher incidence of sex chromosome disomy or nullisomy than by the ICSI technique itself.

Recently, some case reports have mentioned the occurrence of pregnancies after ICSI with spermatids, which are haploid germ cells that may be recovered from wet preparations of testicular biopsies or from ejaculates of azoospermic men. It appears, thus far, that the success rate in terms of fertilization and implantation is rather limited[6]. The use of immature germ cells for ICSI raises concerns related to genomic imprinting, which is the reprogramming of paternal DNA during spermatogenesis. However, in the human it is not known at which stage this process is completed. Modifications in genomic imprinting are known to be associated with certain cancers, for example Wilms tumor[7].

Before the introduction of ICSI, the main problem for infertile couples suffering from severe male infertility was how to become pregnant. Now, the main question is rather whether they are allowed to reproduce themselves through ICSI or whether they accept the possible risks related to some specific applications of ICSI. Counselling of the candidate couples, screening of candidate fathers and longitudinal follow-up of the babies born have become key issues in the treatment.

Because of the novelty of the clinical procedure and its many unknown aspects, at the introduction of ICSI couples were counselled throughout about the novelty and the risks of the procedure. They agreed to participate in a prospective follow-up study of the pregnancies and the children born, including prenatal diagnosis by chorionic villus sampling or amniocentesis. In ICSI, a male germ cell is directly introduced into the oocyte's cytoplasm and all the physiological steps of fertilization are bypassed. This had led some authors to state that ICSI should still be considered an experimental procedure[8]. Thus, initial concerns that had been raised as to the safety of ICSI were related to the piercing of the oocyte which is normally penetrated by a motile sperm[9]. Concerns were raised that this may lead to an increase in major congenital malformations (which are defined as malformations causing functional impairment or requiring surgical correction). So far, there is no evidence that the incidence of major congenital malformations is higher after ICSI than after conventional IVF or natural conception[10–15].

Many couples, infertile because of severe male infertility, can now be successfully treated with ICSI.

ETHICAL CONSIDERATIONS

A genetic abnormality linked to male infertility can be transmitted to the offspring[16]. In such case of possible harm to the child, the dilemma to be faced is of balancing the interests of the child which might ensue from the embryo replaced *in utero* when the research can be safely applied, against the interests of the couple to whom we have a duty of care and who request fertility treatment.

This does not only mean discussing the possible risks for the child with the future parents, but giving counselling, which is ideally the neutral information and support tool used to enable the prospective parents to weigh the possible risks and give their informed consent to the new procedure. Arguably, an informed decision, with possible informed dissent to the proposed screening, is an ideal which can only be reached when a technique is not considered 'experimental' any more. It has also been argued that non-directive counselling may be very hard to perform[17]. This is, perhaps, exemplified by the fact that all patients in the care of the first ever successful team consented both to prenatal diagnosis and to the follow-up of the children[11,13].

Once the child is born, we face, either as (responsible) parents or as practitioners, the arduous decision whether to observe and follow up those born form the new techniques. This epitomizes the difficulty of singularizing without discriminating.

Risks linked to parental anomalies, including genetic abnormalities, raise the same ethical problems as those of genetic counselling in general, as applied to any couple wishing to reproduce when they know of a possible transmissible defect, but who do not need assisted techniques.

With regard to informing and counselling the future parents, the general ethical dilemmas concerning genetic screening and information have been well rehearsed[18]. Rodota asks the pertinent question: are non-paternalistic forms of individual protection possible, or indeed acceptable by all[19]?

When a technique is in the transitional phase from experimentation to becoming a routinely applied procedure, the process of obtaining consent, and of giving the necessary information to make proper consent or dissent, is arguably even more important than when a technique is routinely available and tested[9].

If any form of discrimination based on genetic constitution is unacceptable on ethical grounds[19], it would be just as unethical to refuse treatment to a couple who do not wish to partake of screening, as it would be to disregard a couple's autonomy[20].

As far as the child is concerned, we face a complex dilemma: is it in the child's interest to be informed, or indeed not be not informed. The follow-up of ICSI children is still limited since the first child was born in January 1992. This close follow-up is the result of the concern to avoid a higher prevalance of anomalies than that which exists in natural conceptions. Are we falling prey to the fantasy of 'the perfect child'? This might be seen by those averse to the technique as a reification of the prospective child who has to be 'the best possible product'. But if antenatal and postnatal screening are used to inform the parents of a possible major malformation, then the dilemma is not new any more. It is similar to the complex emotional and moral decisions which any couple may face with the discovery of such an anomaly whatever the means of conception, and has been already discussed and accepted in many societies which have legalized therapeutic termination of pregnancy.

This does not mean that we may not challenge regular practices already enshrined. Thus, if we consider the definition of major malformation as 'those that have an adverse effect on an individual's health, functioning or social acceptability'[11,12], it may be argued that the role of the medical profession is paramount in the prevention of the first factor, but that the role of a caring society as a whole is to facilitate the functioning and the social acceptability of a child suffering the consequences of a major malformation.

In order to behave responsibly towards future generations, there is a need to follow up the children born after replacement of embryos obtained after ICSI. The mother may also be watched, in order to ensure that no harm has occurred to her, but this does not give rise to any unusual problem, as she is able to give consent, or refuse to participate, like any other adult. As far as the children are concerned, several problems arise: the length of time for which the follow-up may be necessary entails an invasion of the privacy of the family concerned. Furthermore, the older the children, the more inappropriate it becomes to perform any test or observation with the consent or dissent given by their parents, and not by themselves. This is reflected in English law by the notion of the 'Gillick competent child', after a famous case concerning the legality of prescribing contraception to those under age[21]. This is further complicated, however, by the later English court's decision to 'apply a higher tariff for refusing a medical examination or procedure than for consenting to one'[22]. Finally, the English Statute also makes it clear that privacy must be respected. Thus, there is no obligation for the parents to inform their children 'that they may be the product of assisted techniques of conception', the wording of the licensed fertility treatments in the English Act.

The psychological aspects are intricate and demand sensitive handling which legislation may not perhaps always portray, although the opportunity for counselling is mandatory in English law[23].

In conclusion, ICSI is undeniably one of the most important advances in the treatment of male infertility in the last decade. The risks may be serious, as with the possible transmission of cystic fibrosis or less serious, as the transmission of male infertility, and hence the necessity of counselling and informing the prospective parents. The technique will also decrease the need for donor insemination, and thus resolve the double ethical problem of the introduction of foreign genetic material to the parenting couple, and of the many aspects of recruitment and selection of donors.

REFERENCES

1. Palermo, G., Joris, H., Devroey, P. and Van Steirteghem, A. C. (1992). Pregnancies after intracytoplasmic injection of a single spermatozoon into an oocyte. *Lancet*, **340**, 17–18
2. Van Steirteghem, A. C., Nagy, Z., Joris, H., Liu, J., Staessen, C., Smitz, J., Wisanto, A. and Devroey, P. (1993). High fertilization and implantation rates after intracytoplasmic sperm injection. *Hum. Reprod.*, **8**, 1061–6
3. Cummins, J. (1997). Controversies in science: intracytoplasmic sperm injection. ICSI may foster birth defects. *J. NIH Res.*, **9**, 34–8
4. Tournaye, H. and Van Steirteghem, A. C. (1997). Intracytoplasmic sperm injection: ICSI concerns do not outweigh its benefits. *J. NIH Res.*, **9**, 35–40
5. Lissens, W., Mercier, B., Tournaye, H., Bonduelle, M., Férec, C., Seneca, S., Devroey, P., Silber, S., Van Steirteghem, A. and Liebaers, I. (1996). Cystic fibrosis and infertility caused by congenital bilateral absence of the vas deferens and related clinical entities. In Van Steirteghem, A., Devroey, P. and Liebaers, I. (eds.) *Genetics and Assisted Human Conception,* Suppl. 4 to *Hum. Reprod.*, Volume 11, pp. 55–80. (Oxford, UK: Oxford University Press)
6. Tesarik, J. (1997). La fecondation humaine sans spermatozoides. *La Recherche*, **295**, 78–83
7. Tesarik, J. and Mendoza, C. (1996). Genomic imprinting abnormalities: a new potential risk of assisted reproduction. *Mol. Hum. Reprod.*, **2**, 295–8
8. Bui, T. H. and Wramsby, H. (1996). Micromanipulative assisted fertilisation – still clinical research. *Hum. Reprod.*, **11**, 925–6
9. De Jonge, C. J. and Pierce, J. (1996). Rewards and risks of ICSI – what kind of reproduction is being assisted? *Hum. Reprod.*, **10**, 2518–28

10. Bonduelle, M., Hamberger, L., Joris, H., Tarlatzis, B. C. and Van Steirteghem, A. C. (1995). Assisted reproduction by intracytoplasmic sperm injection: an ESHRE survey of clinical experiences until 31 December 1993. *Hum. Reprod. Update,* **1**, CD-ROM

11. Bonduelle, M., Legein, J., Buysse, A., Van Assche, E., Wisanto, A., Devroey, P., Van Steirteghem, A. C. and Liebaers, I. (1996). Prospective follow-up study of 423 children born after intracytoplasmic sperm injection. *Hum. Reprod.,* **11**, 1558–64

12. Bonduelle, M., Wilikens, A., Buysse, A., Van Assche, E., Wisanto, A., Devroey, P., Van Steirteghem, A. and Liebaers, I. (1996). Prospective follow-up study of 877 children born after intracytoplasmic sperm injection (ICSI), with ejaculated epididymal and testicular spermatozoa and after replacement of cryopreserved embryos obtained after ICSI. In Van Steirteghem, A., Devroey, P. and Liebaers, I. (eds.) *Genetics and Assisted Human Conception,* Suppl. 4 to *Hum. Reprod.,* Vol. 11, pp. 131–59. (Oxford, UK: Oxford University Press)

13. Wisanto, A., Magnus, M., Bonduelle, M., Liu, J., Camus, M., Tournaye, H., Liebaers, I., Van Steirteghem, A. C. and Devroey, P. (1995). Obstetric outcome of 424 pregnancies after intracytoplasmic sperm injection. *Hum. Reprod.,* **10**, 2713–18

14. Wisanto, A., Bonduelle, M., Camus, M., Tournaye, H., Magnus, M., Liebaers, I. and Van Steirteghem, A. C. (1996). Obstetric outcome of 904 pregnancies after intracytoplasmic sperm injection. In Van Steirteghem, A., Devroey, P. and Liebaers, I. (eds.) *Genetics and Assisted Human Conception,* Suppl. 4 to *Hum. Reprod.,* Volume 11, pp. 121–30. (Oxford, UK: Oxford University Press)

15. Lissens, W., Sermon, K., Staessen, C., Van Assche, E., Janssenswillen, C., Joris, H., Van Steirteghem, A. and Liebaers, I. (1996). Review: Preimplantation diagnosis of inherited disease. *J. Inher. Metab. Dis.,* **19**, 709–23

16. Morris, R. S. and Gleicher, N. (1996). Genetic abnormalities, male infertility, and ICSI. *Lancet,* **347**, 1277

17. Clarke, A. (1991). Is non directive counselling possible? *Lancet,* **338**, 998–1001

18. *Genetic Screening Ethical Issues* (1993). (London: Nuffield Council on Bioethics)

19. Rodota, S. (1993). Genetics, prediction, individual rights. *Inter. Bioth.,* **4**, 199–203

20. Meschede, D., De Geyter, C., Nieschlag, E. and Hosrt, J. (1995). Genetic risk in micromanipulated assisted reproduction. *Hum. Reprod.,* **10**, 2880–6

21. Gillick v West Norfolk and Wisbech Area Health Authority (1984), on appeal (1986), reversed (1986) 685. In Kennedy, I. and Grubb, A. (eds.) *Medical Law.* (London: Butterworth)

22. Devereux, J. A., Jones, D. P. H. and Dickenson, D. I. (1996). Can children withhold consent to treatment? *Br. Med. J.,* **306**, 1459

23. *Human Fertilisation and Embryology Act 1990.* (London: Her Majesty's Stationery Office)

7

Pre-implantation diagnosis and the eugenics debate: our responsibility to future generations

J. Milliez and C. Sureau

Pre-implantation diagnosis entails an array of biological and medical procedures, which can be subdivided into pre-conception diagnosis and pre-implantation embryology. Its goal is to assess the quality of human gametes before fertilization and of human embryos before implantation. One may then eventually select those deemed suitable for development, as inappropriate gametes or embryos are discarded[1].

Pre-implantation embryology triggers the fear of potential genetic manipulation, and is often considered irrationally to be on the slippery slope to all kinds of criminal eugenics[2]. This practice is, for instance, outlawed in the French bioethics legislation of 1994 which forbids anyone 'to enact a eugenic practice with the aim of organising the selection of persons' and indicates punishment with 20 years in jail (Art 511-1). Other fears concern perversions of heredity, or at least poorly controlled intrusions into the genome of germline cells.

We may therefore ask to what extent pre-implantation diagnosis *per se* lends itself to the liability of eugenic practices (according to the French legal definition), to misuse and potentially damaging applications which could be detrimental to future generations.

Two different techniques of pre-implantation diagnosis are available: pre-conception diagnosis (gamete selection) and pre-embryo biopsy, each with their particular problems.

PRE-CONCEPTION DIAGNOSIS

Gamete selection, or pre-conception diagnosis, currently applies only to oocytes. Selection of spermatozoa, for those bearing X or Y chromosomes, for instance, is not yet reliable and is not currently accepted medical practice. Oocytes, however, are amenable to genetic investigation, especially for the detection of aneuploidy within the context of advanced maternal age[3], which is used in two centers worldwide. Several pre-implantation diagnosis programs focus mainly on the evaluation of oocytes collected after ovarian stimulation and subjected to *in vitro* fertilization (IVF). Biopsy of the first polar body can be performed before fertilization and its chromosomal content analyzed after DNA amplification with the polymerase chain reaction (PCR). If the faulty gene is identified in the polar body, then the oocyte carries the normal allele and is therefore suitable for fertilization. If the polar body is normal, then the oocyte carries the genetic defect and it is discarded. Polar body biopsy, although a safe and technically simple procedure not deleterious to the genome of the oocyte, does not take into account the paternal genome.

Particular ethical comments are relevant to this procedure. Since it occurs before fertilization and embryo formation, it involves neither intervention potentially affecting a future life nor an intrusion into the genome. Therefore, it could be ethically ideal, and above any suspicion of eugenism. This argument, however, can only be made for the oocyte. As soon as the gender of the spermatozoon will be accessible to effective identification compatible with gamete survival, large-scale embryonic sex selection will become practicable under the cover of pre-conception diagnosis. Easy access to pre-conception sex selection by the simple means of insemination of selected spermatozoa would represent an obvious temptation to bias the sex ratio, a result already seen in favor of males by means of antenatal diagnosis followed by termination of pregnancy[4]. It has been argued that in countries where baby girls are still exposed to infanticide in the neonatal period, pre-conception sex selection might be considered as a better alternative, and could therefore be advocated as a lesser evil. This, however, begs the question of education towards sex equality, and is discussed at length in Chapter 5.

PRE-IMPLANTATION DIAGNOSIS

Pre-implantation diagnosis is the procedure of choice performed by most centers. Uterine lavage 5 or 6 days after natural fertilization of embryos has become redundant, as there is no guarantee that all embryos have been collected, with the risk of leaving one to develop as an affected pregnancy. Embryos are therefore obtained by *in vitro* fertilization, and biopsy is usually performed on day 3, on a 6–8 cell embryo. One or two blastomeres are removed. There is a large body of evidence, from animal experiments and from human experience[5], that embryo biopsy does not grossly alter the integrity of the individuals born thereafter. Mice bred after embryo biopsy are able to reproduce normally and give birth to normal offspring. Cases of misdiagnosis were due to PCR amplification failure and not to embryo mosaicism, and reliability has been increased by the addition of fluorescence *in situ* hybridization (FISH) in the case of sexing of the embryo.

A total of 56 normal babies have been born worldwide after genetic pre-implantation diagnosis in the context of maternal age, and several in the context of couples with genetic abnormalities. All have been reported to be healthy at birth[6]. There is still proper concern about their long-term health and the unknown risk of untoward development, even though the follow-up of the first of these babies is reassuring. As for IVF or intracytoplasmic sperm injection, the first attempts at embryo biopsy in the human were conducted without documented safeguards, or awareness of the long-term consequences of these manipulations. How shall we justify this scientific breakthrough if it appears to generate lasting prejudice to future generations? So far the only answer, which is purely empirical, is the normal follow-up of IVF babies[7].

It must also be pointed out that, when a new procedure is discovered, the scientist has the duty not to implant the embryos issued from the first attempts in order to diminish the risk of inducing major deleterious consequences for the potential child. It is wise in such circumstances to examine these first zygotes very carefully, by all possible means. This rule is obviously hardly compatible with some legal limits imposed on embryo research, such as those included in the French legislation (Loi 29-7-94) of July 1994.

The most complex ethical question is in fact not so much the current practice of pre-implantation diagnosis, but rather what might be the consequences of its evolving techniques. For instance, multiple PCR and whole genome amplification with multiple primers allows the exploration of up to eight different genes simultaneously from a single blastomere[8]. There is no foreseeable upper limit to the number of genes that will be accessible to evaluation from one or two blastomeres. Will couples demand, after pre-implantation diagnosis, the assurance of a 'perfect' baby[9]? The definition of perfection is debatable, and raises the question of the satisfactory integration of a child into a society which may be richer for more variety. This question was raised recently by Testart and Sèle[2], who discuss the 'production of survivors of this choice, escapees and obligatory servants of an ideology of performance and exclusion' with the danger of exclusion of handicapped people, and 'a more and more restrictive definition of normality and humanity'. If eugenics is defined by its focus on population, and not individual couples' choice to reproduce or not (a child with cystic fibrosis, for instance), this accusation can be contradicted[9,10].

The serious dilemma in the doctor/patient relationship concerns the reluctance most practitioners would feel when faced with a parental request to exclude, at the time of pre-implantation diagnosis for severe genetic disease, embryos also carrying genes associated with diseases which, although serious, are amenable to treatment, such as diabetes or cardiovascular disease. The problem is still different if the request concerns the BCRA1 gene[11], or Huntington's chorea, conditions for which no efficient therapy exists. Arguably, the same concerns have long burdened all those involved in the decision of performing therapeutic terminations of pregnancy. This semantic problem, of the definition of 'serious' (potential) handicaps, different from extreme conditions at birth which entail such suffering as to make them 'unbearably so awful' in cases of selective non-treatment[12], leads us to question further the gray area between prevention of handicap, avoidance and eradication. Let us therefore contemplate the dilemmas stemming from some techniques that might prevent some cases of therapeutic terminations of pregnancy, such as embryonic or germline gene therapy.

EMBRYO THERAPY

Nuclear transplantation will first be mentioned with regards to mitochondrial DNA diseases, which are rare but severe disorders responsible for rapidly lethal or disabling conditions such as encephalomyopathies, Leber hereditary optic neuropathy, or myoclonic epilepsy. They are due to mitochondrial DNA mutations and are maternally transmitted, but both cytoplasm and nuclear DNA are normal. Mitochondrial gene therapy for these disorders must overcome obstacles that are different from those encountered in the search for effective nuclear gene therapy, but such therapy is not beyond the realm of possibility[13].

Before this practice becomes feasible, one could envisage the transfer of the nucleus of an affected embryo into normal cytoplasm, a simple manipulation. Since cytoplasmic mitochondrial DNA is maternally derived, this 'rescued' embryo would give birth to an individual with two genetic mothers. This very peculiar situation is ethically provocative, but in what sense is it basically different from allogenic organ transplantations or from the genetic chimerism established after allogenic bone marrow transplantation in malignant hematological diseases or hematopoietic stem cell grafting for severe immunodeficiencies?

As cloning is forbidden by several legislations (British HUFE Act, French Loi 29-7-94) gene therapy is in practice the true controversial issue. It covers fetal somatic gene therapy and germline therapy. *In utero* gene transfer and fetal gene therapy are of increasing interest among researchers. *In utero* retrovirus- or adenovirus-mediated gene therapy has been proposed as a novel approach to the treatment of inherited lung diseases such as cystic fibrosis or surfactant protein B deficiency[14,15]. Fetal gene therapy through hematopoietic stem cells or fetal liver stem cells has been attempted to treat severe combined immunodeficiency disease (SCID). Fetal bone marrow transplantation has been performed in at least

14 patients with bare lymphocyte syndrome, β-thalassemia or SCID. There are, however, several serious pitfalls to this technique. The fetal immune and inflammatory response to current recombinant retroviral or adenoviral vectors is a significant barrier to *in utero* gene transfer. Foreign substances can be administered safely and tolerated up to only 18–20 weeks of gestation.

Adenoviral vectors must be administered every 2–3 weeks to maintain exposure of the fetus to the recombinant adenovirus carrying the new gene. Experimentally, many sheep fetuses die soon after the initial administration of the virus for yet unknown reasons. Intra-amniotic injection of vectors is not efficient for *in utero* gene therapy. In addition, although fetal gene therapy is targeted towards somatic cells, it is not known to what extent, if it is applied too early in pregnancy or intraperitoneally, it may affect fetal germline cells[16]. Therefore, at present, fetal gene therapy does not seem to come up to expectations. It is not known whether the time is near for the application of embryo and germline gene therapy[17].

Germline or embryo gene therapy is in principle technically feasible. Transgenesis injects genes into the nuclear DNA, transvection incorporates DNA into the cell through viral vectors or liposomes and electroporation moves genes across membranes through an electrical field. All these techniques, however, remain rather clumsy. Transvection with liposomes incorporates the rescue gene into the cytoplasm and not into the nuclear genome. Realization of a transgenic pronucleus is cumbersome, unsuccessful in more than 90% of attempts and needs many more spare cells to be provided after IVF. Integrating vectors such as retrovirus or adeno-associated viruses insert the new DNA at random into the host genome and do not often lead to efficient expression. Insertional mutagenesis leading to tumor formation is a potential risk, albeit remote, for these retrovirus-based vectors[18].

The best means of definitively replacing a deficient gene would probably be embryonic stem cell injection. Embryonic stem cells are totipotent cells and when they are inserted into the blastocele of an embryo they thrive, multiply and ultimately become an integrated cellular mass large enough to express the substitutive gene efficiently. Human diseases that have been modelled in the mouse by means of embryonic stem cell injection include β-thalassemia, Lesch Nyhan syndrome, Duchenne's muscular dystrophy, sickle cell anemia, Gaucher's disease and cystic fibrosis[19]. The corresponding correction of these conditions in human embryos by such means is a tantalizing challenge. Another possibility could be the performance of *in vitro* modifications of the genetic constituents of male gametes during spermatogenesis[20]. Currently, however, we are not yet ready to perform such techniques, and moral issues first pertain to what is feasible.

ETHICAL ISSUES

Current practices

Some of the problems raised are general and valid for all situations in which novel practices are studied, in particular when children and potentially the next generations are concerned. We have already expressed the need, whenever possible, for animal experiments to precede attempts in humans. We have also pointed out the ethical obligation to study the zygote issued from a new technique. Similarly, it may be considered an ethical imperative to master the procedure in human embryos before any replacement. The parents-to-be should be fully informed of all the potential risks, and precise information should be given regarding the scientific and medical nature of the procedure (e.g. whether it is routine, or still in the process of evaluation, or a research procedure). The possible choices must be clearly explained, particularly pre-implantation diagnosis with its constraints vs. a more classical approach, such as prenatal diagnosis and possible therapeutic termination of pregnancy.

The other important concern is that of the potential harm to the fetus and future child, and relates to the kind of surveillance that, once established prospectively, may give answers to questions of risk and possible long-term consequences of these new procedures. The only way to obtain this information is a close follow-up of the children born after the use of these techniques. This in turn entails recording the birth and follow-up of the children. Here lies the dilemma, linked to the respect of the fundamental principle of confidentiality on behalf of the physicians and of autonomy and right to privacy of the patients.

How intrusive may the scientific enquiry be? More precisely, may one impose mandatory recording of all attempts with the new procedures in a national or regional register? What are the limits of these studies: physical, as well as psychosocial?

Apart from the cost of such long-term epidemiological studies, the dilemma of the psychological consequences of this intrusion, in a field which we precisely want to evaluate from this very point of view, is difficult to solve. Moreover, such a follow-up could involve conflict between a legitimate desire of confidentiality by the parents and the interests of the child, and the need to know and be able to inform other parents. If we are reluctant to organize an exhaustive record of the children issued from these novel techniques, can we get enough unbiased information from carefully selected cohorts or case–control studies? This entails two further difficulties, the avoidance of stigmatization and discrimination, and the source of informed consent (the parents or the children?). Whatever the decision, this presupposes that we are in a position to analyze the files of any given case retrospectively, possibly up to adulthood, a situation forecast in the UK, where the HFEA imposes a minimum duration for keeping all national records of children from assisted reproduction[21].

For future prospects, arguments against embryo or germline gene therapy are numerous and most of them very pertinent[17]. There may be no need for embryonic rescue, since IVF nearly always offers a sufficient number of healthy embryos for transfer to women who are normally fertile. The rescue of affected embryos, however, would offer additional embryos for transfer and increase the chances of pregnancy per cycle of stimulation whenever healthy embryos are scarce, when both parents are homozygous for a recessive trait or when one parent is homozygous for an autosomal dominant trait such as Marfan syndrome or retinoblastoma. Much of the discussion is fuelled by the possibility that artificially designed alterations of the human genome in germline cells after embryo gene therapy would be passed to the succeeding generations. The benefit of transmitting a normal gene could be offset by the risk of inducing untoward mutagenesis or carcinogenesis. Indeed, transgenic insertion of the gene into the nuclear DNA occurs at random and may very well induce dysregulation, repression or activation of sensitive genes, oncogene activators or tumor suppressor genes, or any other unknown regulatory gene. Lack of the ability to forecast these consequences means that, for the time being, the scene belongs more to science fiction than to science, although forecasting problems is the first requirement for avoiding them.

Lack of informed consent by members of future generations to alterations in inheritance is an alleged concern, forgetting perhaps that their very existence was probably only possible thanks to the challenged manipulations. Again the debate as to whether life is always more valuable than non-life has been well rehearsed. Finally, it has to be recalled that alteration of the human genome is not a new story, as widespread medications such as colchicine have the capacity to alter the germline genome, and germline mutations are a permanent threat with the manipulation of nuclear energy for weapons, industrial exploitation or nuclear waste storage. This takes us back to the therapeutic duty of the physician to do no harm (*primum non nocere*). Arguably, we have progressed from times in which little but avoidance of harm was possible to times in which the balance of good and harm is taken into consideration. Whether eugenics, the theoretical improvement of humans after the theory of Dalton, is actually good has of course been an important debate this century, and historical catastrophes[22] have led both to the Nuremberg[23] and Helsinki codes[24] and to the systematic stigmatization of any possible (even benignly intended) transmission of a genetic modification[25].

The eugenics debate

Attempts to improve the genetic potential of a 'selected' group of people are not novel. The practices of Nazi Germany and past experience with the sterilization laws in the USA earlier this century remind us that the worst is possible. But what if resistance to infections, including the human immunodeficiency virus or malaria, could be provided in the form of a gene? Should we not provide those affected by familial cancers with the means to avoid this?

Is the basic philosophy of preconception and pre-implantation diagnosis akin to eugenics, in that it selects gametes or embryos? Applied to individuals, families or ethnic groups affected by inherited diseases, it is similar to the current practice of medical interruption of pregnancy, which carries the same negative conotation, especially when it becomes a strategy aiming at eradicating congenital genetic defects in specific areas as for thalassemia in Sardinia. Both practices are accepted because they entail the benefit of freedom from a specific lethal disease in either (future) individuals or members of a community at high risk of genetic disease, both result in the destruction of the faulty human product of conception and prevent the mourning for a stillborn or the grief of watching the suffering of a disabled child. In most instances unaffected carriers are transferred with the possibility of implantation and pregnancy, and terminations of pregnancy are not performed for such indications. This practice represents a formidable ethical assurance, emphasizing that the goal of pre-implantation diagnosis is medical, destined to protect individuals from serious disease, and not some kind of questionable eugenic public health endeavor for the purpose of producing genetic purity.

This consequentialist argument relies only on the soundness of the intention and on the fact that it is neither obligatory nor imposed without consent, but a personal decision of the couple in every case. If it were not, then it might be accused of eugenics, certainly according to the definition of 'eugenic practices' given in the French legislation.

Where will the new ethical border be set? If we break the taboo and tackle research on germline and embryo therapy, we may be stigmatized by those who believe in the sanctity of life from conception. If we do not, we shall be accused of cowardice and lack of vision by those to whom gene therapy is a critical health issue, for themselves and for their offspring[9]. It seems that this point of view may be acceptable to the authorities in the Catholic Church provided zygotes are obtained not by IVF but by GIFT and uterine lavage[26]. Let us find the appropriate moral and scientific resources to solve this modern dilemma.

REFERENCES

1. Edwards, R. G. (1993). *Preconception and Preimplantation Diagnosis of Human Genetic Disease.* (Cambridge: Cambridge University Press)
2. Testard, J. and Sèle, B. (1995). Towards an efficient medical eugenics: is the desirable always the feasible? *Hum. Reprod.,* **11**, 3086–90
3. Plachot, M. (1996). Preimplantation diagnosis: technical aspects. *Third Symposium on Bioethics,* CBDI/SPK (94) 14. (Strasbourg: Council of Europe)
4. Booth, B., Verma, M. and Singh Beri, R. (1994). Fetal sex determination in Punjab, India: correlations and implications. *Br. Med. J.,* **309**, 1259–61
5. Handyside, A. H., Kontogiani, E. H., Hardy, K. and Winston, R. M. L. (1990). Pregnancies from biopsied human preimplantation embryos sexed by Y-specific DNA amplification. *Nature (London),* **244**, 768–70
6. Soussis, J., Harper, J. C., Handyside, A. H. and Winston, R. L. M. (1996). Obstetric outcome of pregnancies resulting from embryos biopsied for pre-implantation diagnosis of inherited disease. *Br. J. Obstet. Gynaecol.,* **103**, 784–8
7. MRC Working Party on Children Conceived by *In Vitro* Fertilisation (1990). Births in Great Britain resulting from assisted conception, 1978–87. *Br. Med. J.,* **300**, 1229–33
8. Zhang, L., Lui, X., Schmitt, R., Hubert, R., Navidi, W. and Arnheim, N. (1992). Whole genome amplification from a single cell: implication for genetic analysis. *Proc. Natl. Acad. Sci. USA,* **89**, 5847–51
9. Shulman, J. D. and Edwards, R. G. (1996). Preimplantation diagnosis is disease control, not eugenics. *Hum. Reprod.,* **11**, 463–4
10. Vines, G. (1995). Every child a perfect child? *New Scientist,* 25 October, 14–15
11. Handyside, A. H. (1996). Pre-implantation diagnosis today. *Hum. Reprod.,* **11** (Suppl. 1), 139–51
12. Kennedy and Grubb (1989). Selective non treatment of neonates. In *Medical Law, Text and Material,* p. 953. (Oxford: Butterworth)
13. Johns, D. R. (1995). Mitochondrial DNA and disease. *N. Engl. J. Med.,* **333**, 638–44
14. McCray, P. B. (1996). *In-utero* gene transfer – an approach to the treatment of inherited lung diseases. *Mol. Hum. Reprod.,* **2**, 469–71
15. Pitt, B. R. and Robbins, P. D. (1996). Retro-virus mediated gene therapy to fetal lung. *Mol. Hum. Reprod.,* **2**, 467–9
16. Iwamoto, H. S. (1996). The window of opportunity for fetal gene therapy. *Mol. Hum. Reprod.,* **2**, 472–4
17. Fiddler, M. and Pergament, E. (1996). Germline gene therapy: its time is near. *Mol. Hum. Reprod.,* **2**, 75–6
18. Douar, A. M., Themis, M. and Coutelle, C. (1996). Fetal somatic gene therapy. *Mol. Hum. Reprod.,* **2**, 633–41
19. Wivel, N. and Walters, L. (1993). Germ-line modification and disease prevention: some medical and ethical perspectives. *Science,* **262**, 533–7
20. David, G. (1995). Rapport sur le diagnostic genetique et la therapie genique. *Bull. Acad. Nle Med.,* **3**, 615–76
21. Human Fertilisation and Embryology Authority (1995). *Code of Practice.* (London: Human Fertilisation and Embryology Authority)
22. Leaning, J. (1996). War crimes and medical science. *Br. Med. J.,* **313**, 1413–15
23. (1947). Nuremberg code. *Br. Med. J.,* **313**, 1448
24. (1964). Declaration of Helsinki. *Br. Med. J.,* **313**, 1448–9

25. Robertson, J. A. (1992). Ethical and legal issues in preimplantation genetic screening. *Fertil. Steril.*, **57**, 1–12
26. Third Symposium on Bioethics (1996). CBDI/8PK. Council of Europe, Strasbourg, France

8

Multiple pregnancies and embryo reduction: ethical and legal issues

I. Nisand and F. Shenfield

INTRODUCTION

In the last ten years, there has been a progressive increase in the incidence of multiple pregnancies of a high order (three or more) in all industrialized countries as a result of the increased use of (super)ovulation induction and assisted reproduction techniques. The untoward effects of these multiple pregnancies stem from both the consequent prematurity of the babies born and the psychological upheaval for the parents[1,2].

Embryo reduction has slowly been accepted and recognized as a medical means of preventing these complications. This efficient and usually safe technique results in (mostly twin) pregnancies whose prognosis is practically identical to that of naturally occurring twin pregnancies. The reduction may fail, however, like any other therapeutic measure, and lead to a complete abortion, with the serious psychological consequences this may entail.

The rationale of the reduction stems from a 'consequentialist' approach (or the lesser of two evils) in which both parents and practitioner balance the benefits and risks from either keeping or reducing a high multiple pregnancy. This cost/benefit analysis is clear in the case of quadruplet (and higher order) pregnancies, in term of both mortality and morbidity, but it is still difficult in the case of triplet pregnancies, for which the most convincing argument is the psychosocial stress endured by the family concerned. In view of the psychological dimensions of the procedure, and of its possible consequences, even if fetal reduction diminishes several of the risks inherent in multiplicity, it cannot be considered a good solution and all efforts should be made to avoid multiple pregnancies.

Prevention is indeed the key word, and has been the motivation behind legislation for instance in the UK in the case of assisted reproduction treatments. Since the passing of the Human Fertilisation and Embryology (HUFE) Act 1990 and the inception of the Human Fertilisation and

Embryology Authority *Code of Practice*[3], which forbids the replacement of more than three embryos in an *in vitro* fertilization (IVF) cycle, the incidence of multiple pregnancies of a high order (quadruplets or more) resulting from such treatment has decreased, and there were none in 1991 resulting from IVF–embryo transfer (ET). There is no restriction, however, on the number of ova replaced in the Fallopian tube in gamete intra-fallopian transfer (GIFT) (unless donation is involved or the procedure is performed in a licensed center), or in the number of follicles stimulated in ovulation induction or controlled superovulation, although many specialist units in the UK have evolved their own sets of guidelines for good practice, in order to avoid multiple pregnancies.

The ethical aspects of the procedure are paramount, and two-fold. First, are those aspects linked to the intrinsic problems of termination of pregnancy which have been discussed from time immemorial in all societies, and have been translated into legislation reflecting the more modern tolerance of the procedure in the latter part of the 20th century. In the UK, the Abortion Act 1967, as modified by the HUFE Act 1990, is still a defense against the Infant Life (Preservation) Act 1929. In France, there is no specific legal disposition on embryo reduction; therefore it is impossible even to assess the number of procedures performed in the country, as they are not included in the obligatory records of both voluntary and therapeutic terminations of pregnancy (Loi sur l'interruption volontaire de grossesse 1975, adopted 1979).

The second aspect, intrinsic to the reduction rather than the termination of pregnancy, revolves around the conflict of interest between the mother-to-be or potential parents and the 'fetal siblings'[4], and will be discussed here.

The intensity of feelings aroused by the procedure has been exemplified by the semantic arguments around its denomination. 'Selective birth' was the term used to describe the outcome of a selective twin termination in a case of abnormality, in 1981[5]. Later, this procedure was respectively called 'selective termination' in English-speaking countries, and 'selective abortion' or 'selective feticide' in France. The term 'selective reduction' was later proposed by Berkowitz and colleagues[6] in order to distinguish it from a selective termination because of an abnormal fetus in a multiple pregnancy. When the only criterion is not a malformation but an excess number of fetuses, there is neither choice nor selection, as the only criterion of choice is the accessibility of the fetus; indeed, the reduction is generally performed at the 11th week, when little is known of either the morphology or the karyotype of the fetus. Therefore, the terms embryo reduction or multiple pregnancy reduction are more accurate. The latter was chosen by the American College of Obstetrics and Gynecology in 1991[7], and applies to all cases in which reduction is performed on one or more apparently normal fetuses in order to reduce the risk of prematurity for the remaining fetuses in the same uterus.

In order to establish a rationale for the reduction, it is essential to analyze the published evidence concerning the risks of multiple pregnancies.

RISKS OF MULTIPLE PREGNANCIES

Natural history of triple and quadruple pregnancies: prematurity

A recent review[8] showed that the average duration of pregnancy for triplets in 707 pregnancies was 33.5 weeks, with 24% born before 33 weeks (definition of severe prematurity), and that 8% were born before 28 weeks. Corrected perinatal mortality for 1000 triplets of more than 500 g was 119 (range 22–312). The corresponding figures for quadruplets from 103 pregnancies were 31 weeks, 45% and 12%, respectively. The frequency of multiple deliveries has increased in 25 years from 0.9% to 1.3% for twins and from 0.9 to 3.7 per 10 000 for triplets[9]. The rise is due both to the increasing age of women at conception, and to the efficacy of the new assisted conception methods.

An American study of 140 triplet pregnancies showed that only 5.7% were the result of spontaneous conceptions[10]. The abortion rate before 24 weeks was 20.7% in the 106 women who did not choose selective reduction, whilst it was 8.7% in the 34 who chose reduction to twins. In France, fertility treatments were responsible for 25% of twin pregnancies and 75% of triplets pregnancies[9]. It is estimated that about 25% of severely premature births come from multiple pregnancies and 9% from fertility treatments.

In IVF, the proportion of multiple pregnancies depends on the age of the mother, the number of embryos transferred, the fertilization rate and the initial diagnosis. There was an incidence of 23.5% of twins (5914 births) and 3.3% of triplets (1319 births) in France resulting from IVF between 1986 and 1994. This was accompanied by 2.4% of embryo reduction, representing 404 reductions in the 16 987 registered pregnancies. Although the average number of embryos transferred per cycle has steadily decreased (2.61 in 1995), there were still 16.2% of transfers of more than three embryos.

Outside IVF, the number is not accurately known, and can be estimated only as a function of the sales of gonadotropins (2.4 million per year in France). It may be possible in France to halve the number of premature births resulting from ovulation induction by reducing respectively by 75% and 30% the number of triplet and twin pregnancies.

Prognosis of severe prematurity

The frequency of the complications of prematurity (cerebral palsy and mental handicap, convulsions, blindness and mental retardation) is a function of the degree of prematurity and of the number of babies born, which means that the same family may have several babies affected by several handicaps after a multiple pregnancy[8]. Babies born between 28 and 32 weeks have a survival rate of almost 80%, but 20% suffer neurological sequelae.

A French study in 1995[11] showed that 15% of premature births came from multiple pregnancies. Severely premature babies (before 33 weeks) were found in 7% of twins and 25% of triplets. Between 25 and 32 weeks of gestation, survival at 2 years increased from 75% to 83% from 1985 to 1992, with an incidence of 13–14% of serious pathologies in the survivors. Scandinavian handicap registers[12] show an increased prevalence of cerebral palsy at 0.24%, similar to rates recorded 40 years ago; this varies between 0.14% for term babies and 8% for extremely premature babies, with 5.4% for premature and 0.8% for moderately premature babies.

Risks of embryo reduction

Embryo reduction was first described in 1986[13], and its full consequences are still under evaluation. The results of an international collaborative study[14] on selective reduction to twins showed identical results after the transabdominal or transvaginal procedure: 84% of pregnancies reached a gestational age of ≥ 33 weeks. The average rate of complete abortion after this invasive procedure, however, is of the order of 8–9%, keeping in mind the 27% rate of spontaneous abortions before 20 weeks in IVF pregnancies. Whilst studies show a correlation between a lesser rate of abortion and the experience of the practitioner, it is impossible to estimate the relative importance of this. In a series of 400 patients undergoing selective reduction published by Mount Sinaï Hospital[15], the results in terms of premature deliveries were better than those expected for the natural history of triplet pregnancies: amongst 179 patients undergoing reduction to twins or singleton, 57% delivered after 36 weeks and 35% between 32 and 36 weeks.

It is uncertain, however, whether this improves the neonatal outcome, as there are few published studies, and they have involved small numbers only[16–18]. There appears to be an increase in birth weight and increased gestational age in reduced pregnancies, a decrease in perinatal mortality, respiratory complications and intraventricular hemorrhage, but there is no evidence of improvement in the long-term prognosis of the survivors. These incomplete results may, however, form the core of the information given to future parents and constitute an argument for the continued availability of embryo reduction in triplets.

Social and familial complications of multiple births

These are serious consequences at the familial level, both for the mother, who finds it difficult to care simultaneously for three children, and for the couple. For the mother, fatigue and stress due to inadequate ancillary or father's help compound the isolation resulting from practical difficulties, and may lead to exasperation and hostility towards the children. Guilt and frustration may result in detachment and lack of enjoyment of the mother–child relationship, especially after the intense yearning for pregnancy.

The couple may find it difficult to adjust to the sudden increase in family size; divorces are not unusual in the first year, and 25% of women need psychotherapeutic help[2]. This study showed three times as many cases of depression 5 years after delivery in mothers of twins as compared to mothers of singletons.

ETHICAL PROBLEMS IN EMBRYO REDUCTION

If embryo reduction is admissible, the notion of 'selection' still presents a particularly difficult problem, especially when one is selecting out a potentially normal fetus. Not only are we dealing with a conflict between the interests of the mother-to-be or potential parents and the fetuses, but also among 'fetal siblings' (Abortion Act 1967). Arguably this selection is in conflict with the notion of justice, which requires us to treat all persons equally according to their needs, and which can be extended to the equal opportunity for life of any single fetus. The practitioner has a duty of care to the couple undergoing fertility treatment (whether 'assisted' or not), and of consideration of 'the welfare of the (potential) child' (a statutory duty under the HUFE Act 1990). It is difficult to reconcile this duty of care to all potential parties with the process of 'reducing' one (or more) of them.

If deontology fails us in this analysis, we may use the consequentialist logic, based on the facts outlined above, in order to analyze the different dilemmas according to the size of the multiple pregnancy. This leads us to consider the reduction of multiple pregnancies in turn according to the number of fetuses.

Multiple pregnancies of a high order (more than three fetuses)

In this case, because of the risk of complete abortion before 24 weeks, the risks of cerebral palsy, the maternal risks and the complications couples have to face when suddenly becoming parents of a large family, the rationale for fetal reduction stems from what Berkowitz and co-workers called 'the life boat argument'[8]. In this analogy, it is acceptable to refuse access to the life boat to people in danger of drowning if the boat is already filled to maximum safe capacity, and to accept them would prejudice other human lives. This is a 'lesser of two evils' argument, in which essential questions still remain: may one life be considered to be more worthy of protection than another, and is it acceptable to abort one seemingly normal fetus to improve the outcome for another?

It is likely that such therapeutic accidents cannot be totally avoided, even with the controls already in place (legislation in IVF, for instance, as is the case in the UK, or professional codes). Therefore, couples undergoing treatment must be informed of the possibility of multiple pregnancy and embryo reduction, even if the practitioner may invoke a conscience clause for the termination. Such a practitioner might be considered unreasonable if he/she were not prepared to assume the consequences in person, but would be legally liable if no information were given. This probably applies both in French law, where there is liability for not fulfilling the duty of care with the legal responsibility involved (in case of complications due to multiple pregnancies), and in English law, where a practitioner may invoke a conscience clause in terminations, but must refer to a colleague who does not have the same qualms.

Twin pregnancies

This case will be used as a paradigm to analyze the differences between termination of pregnancy and embryo reduction, especially in the context of the French legislation, which differentiates between *interruption volontaire de grossesse* (IVG), which is at the mother's request up to 12 weeks, and *interruption therapeutique de grossesse* (ITG) for which there must be a medical indication. In English law, a paragraph of the Abortion Act 1967 (as modified by the HUFE Act 1990) states that 'foetal/embryo reduction' may be lawfully performed if any (other) ground (from S1) applies which relates to a risk to the mental or physical health of the mother that is greater if the pregnancy is continued than if it is terminated. In the summer of 1996, when a case of twin reduction to singleton in the UK was widely discussed in the lay press, Berkowitz argued in a leader in the *British Medical Journal*[19] that, logically, 'if psychological stress is accepted for terminating singletons, it ought to be for reducing twins as well'. But if there is no medical indication, the equating with a singleton termination is not quite accurate. The difference is two-fold: first the reduced pregnancy will continue, albeit in a modified fashion, and is neither terminated nor interrupted; and this very pregnancy is wanted, but not quantitatively so. The embryo is in danger of becoming a commodity, where quantity is as important as quality. As for the parents, any couple planning a pregnancy has a risk of twins of about 1%. Therefore, in the majority of cases, the expectation of twins is not a pathological event. Even though some couples might argue that the technique should be made available in order to have the number of children corresponding to their initial project, one may wonder whether this does not belong more to consumerism on their part rather than to the medical activity of curing and preventing.

In French law, it is legal to terminate a pregnancy up to 12 weeks on request (IVG), which corresponds to the loosely called 'distress' clause of English law. There are, of courses, circumstances in which a twin reduction is medically warranted (malformation of the uterus, previous rupture). The distress of a woman requesting an IVG cannot be compared to the disquiet of a woman who finds herself expecting twins rather than a singleton. It would therefore be advisable to seek the expert advice of counsellors, an obligatory step in ITG in French law, in which the woman's request is not sufficient. This would be in a multidisciplinary setting, in order to assess the appropriateness of the decision of a medical reduction, a process similar to that required in any other case of medical termination.

Therefore, it seems difficult to justify reduction in twin pregnancies, unless there is a medical indication. Otherwise, in itself, it should not be used as an excuse for a couple to avoid a complete termination (IVG), which is a legal possibility up to 12 weeks.

Triplet pregnancies

Between the extremes of high-order multiples and twin reduction, the ethical considerations in the case of triplet pregnancies are most complex. In view of the uncertainties concerning the long-term prognosis in relation to the small difference in prematurity with twins or triplets, it is difficult to perform a cost/benefit analysis on the model of high multiples. As long as indecision prevails on the chances of giving birth to infants in good health, the practitioner's duty is to inform the couple fully of the available evidence on the risks of prematurity, abortion before 24 weeks and the material, psychological and marital stress the couple may face as parents of triplets. They can thus make an autonomous and informed decision.

Minimal invasion is advisable with reduction to twins rather than singleton, in view of the risk of death of one of the twins after a reduction from three to two, whether as a natural complication or a direct consequence of the procedure. Furthermore, the same logic applies as is outlined above concerning the reduction of a twin pregnancy and the reification of the fetus.

CONCLUSION

The medical, psychological and moral implications of embryo reduction are numerous and weigh heavily on the perception of the technique. These cannot be ignored, as it is unlikely that even increased preventive measures, including a statutory framework for ovulation induction, will totally obviate the need to consider such a procedure.

It may be appropriate to set up a framework comparable to the voluntary systems of assisted reproduction treatments (Voluntary Licensing Authority, Fecondation in Vitro Nationale), in order to analyze and audit the use and results of human menopausal gonadotropin therapy. The aim would be to be more cautious with the dosage in ovulation induction, resist the pressure of some patients who are keen for 'prompt intervention' and the temptation to treat early some relatively fertile women who are by nature more at risk of overstimulation. Embryo reduction ('if we have too many, we will reduce') would thus be considered less easily as a routine complementary therapy of assisted reproductive treatment, and the price to pay for efficiency and speed of the expected result, a pregnancy.

Further, to set up embryo reduction within the framework of medical terminations of pregnancy, as it is in English law, with the ensuing obligation of assessment in a multidisciplinary center, would add a downstream check to the upstream prevention. The transparent public statistics of the incidence of reduction would surely be the most efficient strategy to ensure that this technique remains extraordinary rather than routine. It would regain its place, that of a procedure with both grave implications and a psychological cost, like any termination of pregnancy, which is envisaged lightly neither by the couple nor by the medical team.

In spite of our feelings that the reduction of twins to singleton is difficult to justify, and that that of high-multiple pregnancy is difficult not to justify, the most difficult decision remains the case of triplets (even more complex than the case of monozygotic twins and singleton pregnancy). It is here even more essential that the moral standpoint of the practitioner gives way to the responsible decision of the informed future parents, already submitted to iatrogenic trauma. Surely, the crucial words in embryo reduction are 'let us prevent' and 'it is not a routine procedure'.

REFERENCES

1. Petterson, B., Nelson, K. B., Watson, L. and Stanley, F. (1993). Twins, triplets, and cerebral palsy in births in Western Australia in the 1980s. *Br. Med. J.*, **307**, 1239–42
2. Garel, M. and Blondel, B. (1992). Assessment at 1 year of the psychological consequences of having triplets. *Hum. Reprod.*, **7**, 729–32
3. Human Fertilisation and Embryology Authority (1995). *Code of Practice*. (London: Human Fertilisation and Embryology Authority)
4. Rodeck, C. H. (1987). Selective feticide. In Chervenak, F. A., Isaacson, G. C. and Campbell, S. (eds.) *Ultrasound in Obstetrics and Gynaecology*, pp. 1333–8. (Boston: Little, Brown)

5. Kerenyi, T. D. and Chitkara, U. (1981). Selective birth in twin pregnancy with discordancy for Down's syndrome. *N. Engl. J. Med.*, **304**, 1525–7

6. Berkowtiz, R. L., Lynch, L., Chitkara, U. *et al.* (1988). Selective reduction of multifetal pregnancies in the first trimester. *N. Engl. J. Med.*, **318**, 1043–7

7. Committee on Ethics (1991). *Multifetal Pregnancy Reduction and Selective Fetal Termination*, ACOG Committee Opinion No 94, pp. 1–3. (Washington, DC: American College of Obstetrics and Gynecology)

8. Berkowitz, R. L., Lynch, L., Stone, J. and Alvarez, M. (1996). The current status of multifetal pregnancy reduction. *Am. J. Obstet. Gynecol.*, **174**, 1265–72

9. De Mouzon, J. (1996). *Assistance médicale à la procréation et grande prématurité.* (Expertise collective 'Grande Prematurité' Inserm Paris, 1997)

10. Lipitz, S., Reichman, B. N., Uval, J. *et al.* (1994). A prospective comparison of the outcome of triplet pregnancies managed expectantly or by multifetal reduction to twins. *Am. J. Obstet. Gynecol.*, **170**, 874–9

11. Fédération Inserm (1995). *Enquéte périnatale.* (Paris: Fédération Inserm)

12. Hagberg, B., Hagberg, G., Olow, I. and Wendt, L. V. (1996). The changing panorama of cerebral palsy in Sweden, VII, Prevalance and origin in the birth year period 1987–90. *Acta Pediatr. Scand.*, in press

13. Dumez, Y. and Oury, J. F. (1986). Method for first trimester abortion in multiple pregnancy. *Contrib. Gynecol. Obstet.*, **15**, 50–3

14. Evans, M. I., Dommergues, M., Wapner, R. J. *et al.* (1993). Efficacy of transabdominal multifetal pregnancy reduction: collaborative experience among the world's largest centers. *Obstet. Gynecol.*, **82**, 61–6

15. Berkowitz, R. L., Lynch, L., Lapinski, R. and Bergh, P. (1993). First-trimester transabdominal multifetal pregnancy reduction: a report of two hundred completed cases. *Am. J. Obstet. Gynecol.*, **169**, 17–21

16. Macones, G. A., Schemmer, G., Pritts, E. *et al.* (1993). Multifetal reduction of triplets to twins improves perinatal outcome. *Am. J. Obstet. Gynecol.*, **169**, 982–6

17. Boulot, P., Hedon, B., Pelliccia, G. *et al.* (1993). Effects of selective reduction in triplet gestation. *Fertil. Steril.*, **60**, 497–503

18. Lipitz, S., Reichman, B. N., Uval, J. *et al.* (1994). A prospective comparison of the outcome of triplet pregnancies managed expectantly or by multifetal reduction to twins. *Am. J. Obstet. Gynecol.*, **170**, 874–9

19. Berkowitz, R. (1996). From twin to singleton. *Br. Med. J.*, **313**, 373–4

9

Interfaces of assisted reproduction ethics and law

B. M. Dickens

Law and ethics operate in unavoidable interaction with each other as different systems of normative ordering that sometimes overlap and sometimes conflict. For some purposes, they are brought into deliberate intersection, such as when legislation is employed to enforce an ethical value and foreclose the legal choice of ethical error, and when law is challenged on the ground that it produces or, worse, compels, unethical behavior. At first view, law may appear a more powerful instrument than ethics, because its provisions are more authoritatively and accessibly stated by political legislatures and courts, more publicly and systematically exposed, more practically enforceable by legal professional and police officers, more institutionally appealable and more instrumentally changeable. As against this, however, law that is considered to lack an ethical dimension, to be at best crudely pragmatic and at worst ethically bankrupt, is impoverished in its capacity to educate and inspire those it governs to distinguish right conduct from wrong. Law frames the setting within which ethical choices may be practically exercised, but ethics frames the limits within which law is voluntarily obeyed and respected as an expression of the values of the society in which it applies.

The contributions that ethics should make to law and legal process, and the appropriateness of resolving ethical conflicts by law, are matters of continuing social debate. Current debate generated by the expanding range of medical techniques available to assist human reproduction echoes the debate four decades ago in the English-speaking world and beyond, triggered by the Wolfenden Committee Report[1]. Concerned with prostitution and homosexuality, the Report addressed sex not directed towards reproduction, but its discussion of relations between law and morality is equally applicable to medical reproductive technology, which is often directed towards reproduction without sex. Ethics and morality are distinguishable[2], but they are frequently treated as the same, and that practice is followed here.

The Report favored the moral neutrality of law, seeing law as a pragmatic instrument concerned with practical outcomes rather than inherent motivations. Morally flawed conduct may accordingly be accommodated, provided that the conduct and its consequences do not exceed the limits of popular tolerance. The Report rejected an opposing view, namely that law must not only conform to minimum moral standards, but also be employed to enforce and police moral conduct[3] since 'the suppression of vice is as much the law's business as the suppression of subversive activities' (pp. 13–14).

Different legal systems reflect different interactions of law and ethics[4]. Systems reflecting the Anglo-Saxon common law tradition are based on customary practices within their communities. They authorize judges to distinguish between individuals' capacity to act as they wish and their duties to respect the interests of others. The ethical principle of justice that like cases be treated alike has introduced the concept of binding precedent, but legislature may change common law precedents in order to give effect to evolving ethical values. Judges may invoke ethical principles in their reasoning, but the law and legislation are usually regarded as morally neutral and often permit conduct that may be considered immoral. The conditioning approach is that conduct is permitted unless an opponent can show that it violates a law declared by the courts or legislation.

In contrast, civil law reflecting the legal tradition of Continental Europe since the Code Napoléon of 1804 locates all rights in a comprehensive national code that governs all legal claims. Any claimant to a right must first answer the question of where the right is contained within a provision of the code[5], since no legal right can exist outside the code. However, international human rights laws may now establish legal claims outside the terms of national codes. Continental codes often show strong influences of moral values, since historically they were developed under the guidance of religious teachings. A third type of legal system is founded directly on religious law, such as Islamic law. In religious legal systems some regulatory provisions are secular, such as concerning road traffic and industrial pollution, but all laws fit within a religious framework set by spiritual authorities according to their religious texts and inspiration.

These various legal systems shape how laws approach medically assisted reproduction. In common law jurisdictions, such practices as *in vitro* fertilization (IVF) and surrogate motherhood have been initiated without legal restraint, but practices that have come to be considered unethical and intolerable, such as the entrepreneurial promotion of commercial surrogate motherhood agreements, have been restricted by legislation (see, for example, the UK Surrogacy Arrangements Act 1985). In French law in contrast, for instance, a widow's request to receive sperm that her husband had deposited with a banking facility before receiving chemotherapy required her to show under which provision of the Civil Code she could claim sperm that she intended to use for posthumous conception of her deceased husband's child. The sperm bank felt entitled on moral grounds to refuse to give her the sperm[6]. Under Islamic legal systems, for instance, IVF is generally lawful, but only for a wife's pregnancy through her living husband's sperm. Sperm donation by another man is religiously considered unethical as a sin falling short of adultery, and is unlawful regarding married or unmarried women[7].

The overwhelming majority of techniques of assisted reproduction raise the issue of whether their employment should be governed by laws, or be left to individual, professional or institutional ethical judgment. Discrimination on grounds of race, religion and, for instance, sex, tends to be legally condemned according to human rights laws applied at international and national levels[8], but reproductively impaired people have not customarily been regarded as specially susceptible to unlawful discrimination. Legislation is usually proposed in order to restrict access to means of assisted reproduction rather than to promote equitable access. Similarly, the needs of infertile people whose childbearing might be facilitated through embryo research tend to be discounted in arguments opposing such research on grounds of the moral status of the zygote and embryo. The view that embryos should not deliberately be created only for research, but that research may be undertaken if at all only on 'spare' embryos left for instance from IVF procedures, equally discounts the claims of infertile patients.

Decisions showing conflicts between ethical principles applied at the individual (or microethical) level and at the social (or macroethical) level are particularly problematic for embodiment in law. The issue of abortion remains contentious, but legal systems increasingly recognize the decision to be that of the individual woman, at least at the earlier stages of pregnancy[9]. However, those usually protective of individual women's microethical right of choice may experience conflict regarding abortion on grounds of fetal sex. Even where evidence shows no general preference for male rather than female children (in Canada, for instance[10]), sex selection techniques may be opposed because they could be used to abort female fetuses, and so perpetuate a perception of women's inferiority and the devaluation of girl children.

Individual choice supported at the microethical level may be opposed at the macroethical level of sex selection, on symbolic grounds. However, legal prohibition of the microethical option in the absence of empirical evidence of its social harm 'would risk eroding other aspects of women's reproductive autonomy' (reference 10, p. 916). Prohibition of disclosure of fetal sex denies autonomy both to terminate the pregnancy of a fetus of a disfavored sex, and, to a woman whose family is complete and who is disposed to terminate an unplanned pregnancy, to continue if the fetus is of a favored sex.

Ethical guidelines, codes and proposals for conducting research and delivering services to assist reproduction have been developed by a wide range of social and medical bodies, including those constituted by governmental, intergovernmental, professional and specialist agencies. Some primarily address matters of technique, such as limits on how many pre-embryos may be placed *in utero*, indications for fetal reduction and biological criteria for use, donation and preservation of gametes and pre-embryos. Others address how laws should respond to assisted reproduction, for instance whether presumptions of parenthood and rights to child custody should be governed by criteria of gamete supply, gestation, social intent or children's best interests. Solutions preferred among ethical choices frequently vary, and some are inconsistent with others. For instance, some consider a woman should serve as a gestational ('surrogate') mother only if she has previously delivered a child because only she can give truly informed consent to pregnancy and childbirth. Others consider that no woman rearing a child should serve in this role, lest the child may feel threatened on learning that she was willing to surrender a child to another person.

Ethical guidelines proposed by professional and specialist agencies that are not afforded the direct force of law by legislation may nevertheless be given legal effect indirectly. Courts identifying standards of reproductive practice and counselling below which legal negligence will be found may approve guidelines proposed by such agencies as furnishing the content of legal standards. Contracts for services that professionals make with their patients or clients may be judicially interpreted to import ethical guidelines by which such professionals profess to be bound. Failure to observe them will then in law constitute breach of contract. Further, practitioners contractually engaged in hospital or other clinics may be found in breach of their contractual agreements for disregard of such guidelines. Professional licensing authorities may similarly consider disregard a disciplinary offence, and impose sanctions for professional misconduct or unethical behavior, such as license withdrawal or suspension, that courts of law will uphold. When health care practitioners and counsellors are required to observe ethical guidelines by courts that set standards of care in negligence law, for compliance with private contracts and for retention of licenses permitting public practice of legally regulated health or associated professions, the guidelines acquire significant legal enforcement and influence.

The conversion of ethical guidelines into law by legislation that introduces criminal punishment for violation may represent the integration of ethical and legal principles, but it may also be harmful to the promotion of ethical reflection and decision-making. Laws that seem to reinforce ethical conduct may actually replace the exercise of ethical judgement with unreflective obedience to law. If the nature and consequences of ethical misconduct in assisted reproduction are considered so harmful that such misconduct cannot be tolerated or risked in a society, it may be deterred by legislation aimed to secure behavioral compliance. If a society wishes to promote the exercise not of mere obedience to a legally enforced code of conduct but of responsible ethical judgement, however, it must be tolerant of choices within a range of ethical options, including some that even a majority of its members consider erroneous or flawed.

Law may compete against ethics as the decisive influence in conduct, and prevail at the cost of ethics. A population may come to obey law under the threat of legal punishment but cease to practice and understand ethical judgment. Laws enforced through the menace of punishment that once rested on moral inspiration and virtue may come to be based only on the fact of power. Such law may accordingly fail to educate society on the distinction between ethical and unethical behavior, and teach only the cynical, morally impoverished lesson that might is right. The urge to use law to enforce moral conclusions may be pursued at too heavy a cost to the health of the moral sensitivity and judgment the law was intended to promote. The Wolfenden Report[1] (page 24, paragraph 61) observed that 'there must remain a realm of private morality and immorality which is, in brief and crude terms, not the law's business.'

REFERENCES

1. The Wolfenden Committee (1957). *Report of the Committee on Homosexual Of- fences and Prostitution*, Cmnd. 247. (London: HMSO)
2. Roy, D. J., Williams, J. R. and Dickens, B. M. (1994). *Bioethics in Canada*, pp. 37–8. (Scarborough, Ontario: Prentice-Hall)
3. Devlin, P. (1965). *The Enforcement of Morals*. (Oxford: Oxford University Press)
4. Dickens, B. M. (1994). Legislative approaches to assisted reproduction. *J. Assist. Reprod. Genet.*, **11**, 327–31
5. Baudouin, J. -L. and Labrusse-Riou, C. (1987). *Produire l'homme: De quel droit?* (Paris: Presses Universitaires de France)
6. Trib. gr. inst. Créteil, 1 August 1984, Parpalaix, v. C.É.C.O.S., Gaz. Pal. 1984. II. 560
7. Fayad, M. M. (1992). Ethics in assisted procreation in Egypt. *Popul. Sci.*, **12**, 123–9
8. Brownlie, I. (1983). *Systems of the Law of Nations, State Responsibility*, Part I, p.81. (Oxford: Oxford University Press)
9. Henshaw, S. K. (1992). Induced abortion: a world review, 1990. In Butler, J. D. and Walbert, D. F. (eds.) *Abortion, Medicine and the Law*, pp. 406–34. (New York and Oxford: Facts on File)
10. Royal Commission on New Reproductive Technologies (1993). *Proceed with Care: Final Report of the Royal Commission on New Reproductive Technologies*, pp. 889–917. (Ottawa: Canada Communications Group-Publishing)

10

The views of the patients

C. Ramogida

INTRODUCTION

From the patient's point of view, some ethical dilemmas are voiced more frequently than others, particularly those relating to gamete donation, access to treatment, anonymity and secrecy.

GAMETE DONATION

For the patients, oocyte and sperm donation differ radically in practice, and in spirit. The possibility of cryopreservation in the case of sperm has enormous practical advantages, but recourse to donor insemination (DI) is still very difficult psychologically for the man who finds it hard to separate sexuality and reproduction. Right up to the delivery of the infant produced by DI the question uppermost in the mind of the couple is more 'whom will he/she look like?', rather than 'will he/she be normal?'. Fortunately, in the great majority of cases, the bonding between father and child is immediate. The recent introduction of microinjection techniques has proved, from information of our patients' support group, to be a much favored alternative to DI.

In the case of oocyte donation, we have to face public prejudice which associates the technique with donation to women of 45 years and more. We know that premature menopause and Turner's syndrome are a small proportion of fertility problems, but believe that minorities also have a right to proper treatment.

The fact that anonymity is compulsory in France complicates matters enormously. As acceptable as this principle may be in the case of DI, where sperm can be frozen, some leeway is necessary in the case of oocyte donation.

Knowing of the complexity of oocyte induction and retrieval, many women would donate to their sister, but not perhaps be motivated to give to an anonymous recipient. In recent French legislation, this means for the recipient couple the necessity to consent in front of a judge or notary.

After this, they are given an appointment in a hospital fertility center, even if no donors are available, but a woman over 43 years is excluded. If the couple introduces a donor who would donate to other recipients, the average waiting time of 18 to 24 months may be reduced by about 6 months. If the treatment fails, they will go through the same lengthy wait again.

For these reasons I feel that legislation should be less restrictive as regards anonymity. Furthermore, when it is realized that oocyte recipients feel indebted to the donors, whether or not a pregnancy has been achieved, it is also perhaps time to challenge the principle of unpaid donation.

ACCESS TO TREATMENT

What are the appropriate bodies who might reassess these problems? Twenty years after women used to go abroad in order to obtain an abortion, then illegal in France, other women do the same in order to obtain oocyte donation, because of restrictive legislation in France. This proves that no legislation can ultimately prevent infertile couples from seeking help elsewhere, although of course only those who can afford it will do so. Perhaps this can be avoided, at least in Europe. As far as the patients are concerned, justice must prevail and treatment should be accessible to all, with no difference between rich and poor. It is essential that all who yearn for a child may at least be given hope.

SECRECY

Many papers have been written on the matter of secrecy and anonymity in gamete donation. From my experience as a representative of patients' associations, I am certain that no legislation in the world may dictate to the parents of the children of gamete donation how to behave regarding this matter. After organizing several round-table discussions on the subject, I am aware of the disparity of views, and of their evolution with time and life events. One outcome is that it seems better to inform the child of his/her origins at a young age rather than at adolescence, if this is the path chosen. What is certain, is that parents want to be informed about all the consequences of their treatment on the future of their child, the bad news as well as the good news. And if they are so intent on pregnancy that the welfare of the child becomes secondary, this information must be given even more emphatically.

In conclusion, the end of the 20th century has seen formidable advances in human reproduction. No one knows how much further medical and social progress may advance. Patients' associations are claiming the right of full participation in the hopes for fertility in the 21st century, symbolized by the 200 000 children already born of assisted reproduction. Many of us have renounced privacy for our children, in order that further children of assisted reproduction may become themselves quite ordinary and anonymous. We are part of an experimental generation, which has rapidly shown that it can be an active community, and will continue to inform others with the same needs.

Conclusion

F. Shenfield and C. Sureau

Most people, and especially the couples who have benefited from the techniques of assisted reproduction, and their physicians, are thankful to Steptoe and Edwards[1] for their achievement, research and contribution to *in vitro* fertilization (IVF). A minority regret the sorrow engendered by failure in the face of high technical hopes, the reification of the embryo, the satisfaction of fantastic desires of fertility, and especially the possible worrying consequences on future generations or the hidden eugenics which they claim is the consequence of the derivatives of IVF.

The editors are thankful for all the questions raised, as they prompt us all to challenge many ideas and dogmas.

In some cases we are progressing towards a *de facto* acceptance, if not a real consensus, even if some reserves and uncertainties remain. This is the case for the provision of information and non-directive counselling necessary for informed consent, which represents the respect of the principle of autonomy. Here we must stress that this is not quite identical in French and English, or Continental and Anglo-Saxon philosophies; it is much more individualistic in the latter, but symbolic of a popular will democratically expressed in the former, according to the form of the 'social contract' of J.J. Rousseau. Thus it is in the law, especially Statute law, that we have the basis of an ethical consensus, as explained by Dickens in Chapter 9.

There is almost universal recognition of the necessity for animal research, and of its limits. As for embryo research, there is general agreement to condemn the creation of hybrids, cloning by multiple division of blastomeres and nuclear transfer or parthenogenesis. This also applies to gene therapy, more for practical than theoretical reasons.

The concern for future generations is universal, even if the means of follow-up lead to debate about coercion.

Sex selection for non-medical reasons evokes a great deal of unease, much more than when timing of intercourse or peculiar diets were recommended for this effect. Must we conclude that its tolerance was a function of the inefficiency of those methods?

The principle of non-commercialization is also consensual at a worldwide level (UK, France, AFS, FIGO, Council of Europe), and one for which the editors are well-known proponents. It is modified of course by the inclusion of some assisted reproduction techniques in the private sector, and sometimes the 'just reward' for 'gifts'. In fact, all agree that one must avoid the exploitation of human distress. We chose to print the dissenting voice of Dr Lockwood (Chapter 3), who refers to oocyte donation, which presents a particular problem of scarcity, as outlined in Chapter 10 on behalf of the patients. We hope that several schemes enhancing solidarity will actually be successful.

The eugenics problem, debated about pre-implantation diagnosis, is more controversial. All agree to condemn eugenics leading to the favored or forbidden procreation of individuals sharing some ethnic, physiological or pathological characteristics, either by coercion or enticement. This is different, however, from seeking an individual, voluntary, favorable influence on procreation as it is done, in several countries, with antenatal care. Prenatal diagnosis, leading to the destruction of some potential individuals, may correspond to a 'eugenic' attitude, but is not generally condemned. Is pre-implantation diagnosis a less violent, more subtle and perverse form of eugenics, not so much because of its present results, but more because of its supposed evolution? This is unlikely.

Is germline therapy the fearful epitome of eugenics practices, or an early form of therapy, as described by some Catholic theologians and practitioners, in that it both avoids a disease and avoids its transmission? Finally, is it wrong to practice some techniques which may be at the margin of eugenic practice whilst we facilitate the reproduction of persons who may transmit some genetic abnormalities?

We see that subjects often considered consensual may quickly experience controversy or varied interpretations. Some other fields are even more prone to dissent and controversy:

(1) The anonymity vs. disclosure debate for the children resulting from gamete donation, with the conflict between the secrecy often desired by the parents, and the 'right of the child to know his/her origins' inscribed in the Convention for the Rights of the Child, although this was designed to respond to precise political circumstances. We chose not to include this, as one of the editors has recently been involved in the debate;

(2) Surrogacy, illegal in France, legal and controlled on the UK, and sometimes commercial in the USA;

(3) The legitimacy of the inclusion of fertility treatments in any national health system, and the relationship with social justice and its costs (a political question, if ever there was one);

(4) Embryo reduction, in particular of triplets;

(5) The creation of embryos for research purposes, which if banned would mean the end of studies on gametes (oocyte freezing, sperm washing in case of HIV positivity) as it entails the analysis of the resulting

embryos for safety. Is there any real difference between creating embryos specifically for research, or creating numerous spare embryos so that some are available if necessary? This was pointed out by I. de Beaufort at a recent meeting on the status of the embryo at the Council of Europe; and

(6) Even more esoteric problems, left voluntarily out of the scope of this book, such as the treatment of post (natural) menopausal women with oocyte donation, posthumous fertilization or implantation and sperm collection by electroejaculation in a comatose man.

Problem number 5, of the nature and status of the embryo, is that in which dogmatic positions are most polarized between these who consider the embryo to have an identity of a person, and those who prioritize the autonomy of the woman. This same debate was beautifully analyzed by Dworkin[2] in *Life's Dominion* in the context of abortion, and opposes those against IVF as a matter of principle (the 'ethics of conviction' of Max Weber[3]), and those who sometimes also dogmatically assert autonomy and its market consequences as paramount, like Engelhardt[4].

We must, however, live together in a (hopefully) democratic society, and this is where legislation comes into play. It affords a different protection to the embryo according to circumstances, a gradual protection that corresponds to the notion of a potential person. Legislation, of course, should be loose and tolerant enough not to be the sole vehicle of the prevalent ideology in any society, in order both to protect individual freedom, and to avoid the blunting of personal responsibility. This is easier to achieve in common law systems that with statutes (Chapter 9).

It seems, however, that we are progressing towards a middle way: the UK was first to establish statutory authority in assisted reproduction, and France has asked a special commission to settle the problems stemming from the restrictions on embryo research and 'studies'. This evolution seems necessary when European borders are becoming permeable both to practitioners and to patients and when the European Court of Human Rights may influence national law.

The future path must be the enhancement of the notion of responsibility (described by Hans Jonas) for both practitioners and patients, based on the beneficence which should be the motivation of any medical act and which Levinas[6] called 'kindness of Man towards Man'.

REFERENCES

1. Edwards, R. G., Steptoe, P. C. and Purdie, J. M. (1980). Establishing full-term human pregnancies using cleaving embryos grown *in vitro. Br. J. Obstet. Gynaecol.*, **87**, 737–56

2. Dworkin, R. (1993). The morality of abortion. In *Life's Dominion, An Argument about Abortion and Euthanasia*, pp. 30–68. (London: Harper Collins)
3. Rameix, S. (1996). *Fondements Philosophiques de l'Ethique Médicale*, p. 136. (Paris: Ellipses)
4. Engelhardt, H. T. (1995). Human reproduction: conflicts at the roots of bio-ethics and health care policy. In Sureau, C. and Shenfield, F. (eds.) *Ethical Aspects of Human Reproduction*, pp. 49–61. (Paris: John Libbey)
5. Dworkin, R. (1993). The morality of abortion. In *Life's Domain, an Argument about Abortion and Euthanasia*, p. 14. (London: Harper Collins)
6. Rameix, S. (1996). *Fondements Philosophiques de l'Ethique Médicale*, p. 132. (Paris: Ellipses)

Index